THE 95% VEGAN DIET

WORKBOOK

THE 95% VEGAN DIET

-DIET-

WORKBOOK

JAMIE NOLL, PHARM. D., LD, CDE AND CAITLIN E. HERNDON, JD

TATE PUBLISHING
AND ENTERPRISES, LLC

The 95% Vegan Diet Workbook
Copyright © 2013 by Jamie Noll, Pharm. D., LD, CDE and Caitlin E. Herndon, JD. All rights reserved.

No part of this publication may be reproduced, stored in a retrieval system or transmitted in any way by any means, electronic, mechanical, photocopy, recording or otherwise without the prior permission of the author except as provided by USA copyright law.

This book is designed to provide accurate and authoritative information with regard to the subject matter covered. This information is given with the understanding that neither the author nor Tate Publishing, LLC is engaged in rendering legal, professional advice. Since the details of your situation are fact dependent, you should additionally seek the services of a competent professional.

Disclaimer: Neither the authors nor the publisher are engaging in rendering professional advice or services, medical or legal, to the individual reader. The information provided in The 95% Vegan Diet and The 95% Vegan Diet Workbook is directed towards relatively healthy adults. It is not intended to replace the advice of your personal physician. Anyone who has a medical condition should be under the care of a qualified physician, and all matters of health should be discussed with your physician. If there is any doubt concerning the applicability of any of the information contained within this book, you should discuss the matter with your physician. Neither the authors nor the publisher shall be liable or responsible for any loss or damage allegedly arising from any information or suggestion in this book.

The opinions expressed by the author are not necessarily those of Tate Publishing, LLC.

Published by Tate Publishing & Enterprises, LLC
127 E. Trade Center Terrace | Mustang, Oklahoma 73064 USA
1.888.361.9473 | www.tatepublishing.com

Tate Publishing is committed to excellence in the publishing industry. The company reflects the philosophy established by the founders, based on Psalm 68:11,
"The Lord gave the word and great was the company of those who published it."

Book design copyright © 2013 by Tate Publishing, LLC. All rights reserved.
Cover design by Ronnel Luspoc
Interior design by Caypeeline Casas

Published in the United States of America

ISBN: 978-1-62563-818-2
1. Health & Fitness / Diet & Nutrition / General
2. Cooking / Vegetarian & Vegan
13.07.29

DEDICATION

· ·

We dedicate this workbook to all of our readers.
The power to change the face of things, to create a ripple effect, lies within each of you.

CONTENTS

Introduction 11

The Importance of Learning How to Fish 13

Home-Based Assessments for Nutritional Health Status 15

Laboratory Assessments for Nutritional Health Status 21

The Macronutrients, Water, Fiber, and Organic 39

    Carbohydrate 39

    Fat 42

    Protein 42

Water 45

Fiber 49

Organic or Not? 51

    Dirty Dozen™ 51

    Clean 15™ 52

Reading Labels for Veganism 53

Vegan Frugal Fun by the Season 55

    Spring (March 21–June 20) 55

        Spring's Seasonal Fruits and Vegetables 55

        St. Patrick's Day 58

        Earth Day 60

        Easter 62

Cinco De Mayo 64

Summer (June 21–September 21) 67

    Seasonal Fruits and Vegetables 67

    July Fourth 70

    The Feast of Mother Cabrini (Aug 24–Sept 3) 72

    Labor Day 74

Fall (September 22 - December 20) 77

    Seasonal Fruits and Vegetables 77

    Rosh Hashanah 80

    Oktoberfest 82

    Halloween 84

    Thanksgiving 86

Winter (December 21 - March 20) 89

    Seasonal Fruits and Vegetables 89

    Hanukkah 92

    Christmas 94

    Kwanzaa 96

    New Year's Day 98

    Chinese New Year 100

    Super Bowl Sunday 102

    Mardi Gras 104

    Valentine's Day 106

Exercise and Sleep 109

    Exercise 110

    Sleep 116

Weight Loss 121

Prediabetes and Type 2 Diabetes Mellitus 127

Become Your Own Scientist 131

    What is Good Science? 131

    Diet, Supplements, and Your Prescription and Over-the-Counter Medication 183

Create a Ripple Effect 185

    The First Ten Guidelines to Create a Ripple Effect, Generation to Generation 185

    Your Plan for Creating a Ripple Effect 187

Quit Smoking 189

References 213

    The Importance of Learning How to Fish 213

    Home-Based Assessments for Nutritional Health Status 213

    The Macronutrients: Carbohydrate, Fat, and Protein 214

Index 217

INTRODUCTION

Congratulations! The fact that you purchased this workbook means that you are ready to make a change in your nutritional and overall health. The saying "strike while the iron is hot" is very relevant; learn and make changes while you are highly motivated. This workbook will not only help you get started; it will help keep you focused over the longer haul—five years. The reason we decided to make this workbook span over five years is because, as we mentioned in *The 95% Vegan Diet,* your health is a big picture, not how you feel in a moment or a week or two. It is essentially an average of successfully meeting health goals over many years. Sure, there are outliers in the equation, such as those who had no health issues and then died suddenly and those who abused their health for many years and lived to be one hundred, but the majority of us will fall into the middle ground.

This workbook provides a means for which you can record your results for the *homework* assignments in *The 95% Vegan Diet,* but it is much more. It will help you build upon what you learn over the period of five years, starting from the time you read *The 95% Vegan Diet:* the recipes you have tried, holiday meal plans, a good science checklist, and more. This is, in essence, a five-year journal of your nutritional journey, progress toward health goals, and the progression you put into place for family traditions. It is a new beginning and a systematic plan for your health!

We suggest you keep this workbook with you at all times. You never know when you might learn something that you should record! Also, you will definitely need to bring this book to the appointments with your physicians and other healthcare providers.

Hopefully, what you learn over the next five years will be what you continuously teach your children and grandchildren; create that ripple effect for the generations to come so that they do not suffer the ravages of poor healthcare decisions. In addition, we hope you will become a leader and champion for the health in your community. There are so many outlets for one who is motivated to change the face of things!

We wish you the very best on your journey!

THE IMPORTANCE OF LEARNING HOW TO FISH

"If you give a man a fish you feed him for a day. If you teach a man to fish you feed him for a lifetime."

—Lao Tzu, Fourth Century BC, Chinese Proverb

It is a fact that actively engaging the student in the learning process provides a much greater retention rate.[1] You will likely not retain the teachings in *The 95% Vegan Diet* without somehow being actively involved in your learning. So while it may seem tedious at times to write things out, in five years' time, you will be amazed at how far you have come! Invest in yourself, and don't become frustrated with the work you must put into understanding and being in control of your health. There is truly nothing as important!

"Tell me and I will forget. Show me and I may remember. Involve me and I will understand."

—Chinese Proverb

HOME-BASED ASSESSMENTS FOR NUTRITIONAL HEALTH STATUS

BMI (Body Mass Index) combined with your waist measurement almost always provides a clear picture of your overweight status.[1,2] To calculate your BMI, you can use an online calculator, such as is available on the CDC website: http://www.cdc.gov/healthyweight/assessing/bmi.

You can also calculate your BMI using this equation:

$$BMI = [\text{weight in pounds} \div (\text{height in inches} \times \text{height in inches})] \times 703$$

Or you may prefer to calculate in metric:

$$BMI = \text{weight in kilograms} \div (\text{height in meters} \times \text{height in meters})$$

For example, if a person weighs 200 pounds (90.9 kg) and is 5ft, 6in (1.68 meters) tall, the calculation would be the following below.

Using pounds and inches:

$$[200 \div (66 \times 66)] \times 703 = 32.3$$

Using metric measurements:

$$90.9 \div (1.68 \times 1.68) = 32.5$$

Normal BMI ranges from 18.5 to 24.9, overweight BMI ranges from 25.0 to 29.9, class I obesity ranges from 30.0 to 34.9, class II obesity ranges from 35.0 to 39.9, and extreme obesity is a BMI of 40 or above. In the case above, with a BMI of 32.3, the person would be considered obese class I.

If there is a question of whether BMI is an accurate assessment of weight status, you can measure your waist circumference. To do this, place a tape measure around your abdomen above the hip bones (iliac crests) and over the umbilicus (belly button), as illustrated in figure 1 below. Do not make the tape measure so tight that it indents your skin. Visually check to make sure the tape is at an even height all the way around. For women, if the measurement is 31-1/2 inches or greater, that would signal that the BMI measurement is likely an accurate depiction of weight status. For men, the waist measurement of 37 or above would be a signal that the BMI measurement is an accurate depiction of weight status.

Figure 1

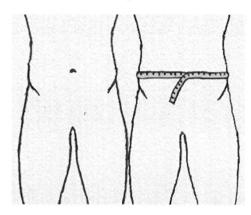

I can't tell you how many patients and people I have spoken to who are critical of BMI and don't think it is appropriate for them. However, the fact is that BMI is appropriate for the majority of people; most simply do not want to face it. You would have to be *extremely* muscular or have an obviously large frame for it not to work for you.

BMI status and waist circumference used together almost always provide an accurate picture for a person's risk for developing chronic and deadly diseases.[1,2] And although the literature cites varying measurements that signaled certain increases in risk status for cardiovascular disease, diabetes, colon, and breast cancer, it is safe to say in general that the greater the waist measurement, the greater the risk.

It is very important to *know* what your goal is in order to *progress toward* your goal. Since your goal should be less than 25, we can calculate what you should weigh in order to attain a BMI of 24.9. You can either go back to the CDC BMI calculator or use the following equations. The equations will tell you what you need to weigh in order to have a BMI of 24.9.

$$\text{weight in pounds} = \frac{[\text{Height in inches} \times \text{Height in inches}] \times 24.9}{703}$$

or

$$\text{weight in kg} = [\text{Height in meters} \times \text{Height in meters}] \times 24.9$$

The following table provides room for sixty BMI entries, one per month for five years.

My weight goal to attain a BMI of 24.9 =		
Date	BMI	Waist Circumference

THE 95% VEGAN DIET WORKBOOK

My weight goal to attain a BMI of 24.9 =		
Date	BMI	Waist Circumference

My weight goal to attain a BMI of 24.9 =		
Date	BMI	Waist Circumference

Body fat measurement is also indicative of overweight/obesity status. However, it is more difficult to ascertain this number, and there are no solid guidelines for what your percentage of body fat should be. Healthy percentages appear to vary and are dependent on other variables, such as sex and ethnicity. There are several ways in which your percentage of body fat can be measured, ranging from measurement of skinfold thickness to ultrasonography. There are machines available on the market for laypersons to measure their own body fat percentage, but the most accurate measurements are performed in metabolic laboratories. If you would like to use any of the available tools to measure your body fat percentage, note that it is not as important to have the precise percentage, but to use that number as a starting point upon which you would like to improve. For example, no matter what tool you choose to use, if your percent body fat comes up as 35 percent, using the same tool you used to get that measurement, you can watch for any improvements relative to the baseline number. Just be sure to use the same measuring device each time so that your relative improvement can be accurately depicted.

The following table provides room for sixty months or five years for tracking your body fat measurements, if desired:

My personal goal of body fat percentage =	
Date	% Body Fat

THE 95% VEGAN DIET WORKBOOK

My personal goal of body fat percentage =	
Date	% Body Fat

My personal goal of body fat percentage =	
Date	% Body Fat

LABORATORY ASSESSMENTS FOR NUTRITIONAL HEALTH STATUS

Taking blood and urine samples are your physician's means to see if there are any signals to be concerned about with your health, with respect to nutritional status, diabetes, cardiovascular disease, and some cancers. (Of course, this does not cover other necessary routine exams, such as mammograms, pap smears, prostate checks, and colonoscopies. These other screenings are outside our scope, so please discuss what you need and how often based on current clinical screening recommendations.) If the basic blood panels are normal, except in rare cases, it tells us that there is nothing further that needs to be tested at that time; you are fine. You have no chronic or deadly diseases. With simple blood and urine samples, the presence or risk of the diseases in question is determined, as well as your nutritional status. The blood tests that should be ordered by your physician include a CBC (complete blood count), a comprehensive metabolic panel, a Vitamin D level, a thyroid panel, a lipid profile, blood sugar (blood glucose) values both fasting and two hours after you have eaten (two hours postprandial), a C-reactive protein (CRP) level and liver function tests. Depending on your age and personal or family history, your physician may also recommend you have an EKG (electrocardiogram) done. He or she may also request other tests due to your previous or family health history. The urinalysis essentially tells your physician if your kidneys are spilling protein and/or glucose. It is abnormal to find either one in the urine. Also, if the urine is unusually dark, it may indicate you are not properly hydrated. Very dark urine sometimes indicates there is blood in it.

Note that I cannot provide exact laboratory values for normal ranges of the various blood tests discussed here, as those values differ from lab to lab. You will see what the normal ranges are for your laboratory on your lab results.

The CBC measures all of the blood cells (red and white blood cells): your hemoglobin and hematocrit, your platelets, and the size of your red blood cells. Among other things, your doctor can determine your immune status, how well your body is prepared to fight infections, or if you have an active infection. It can also signal if you are iron, vitamin B_{12}, or folic acid (another B vitamin) deficient. This test is particularly important for those following a vegan diet because without meat products or proper supplementation, they can become vitamin B_{12} and iron deficient. A B_{12}

deficiency results in a type of anemia, called a macrocytic or megaloblastic anemia. To confirm the diagnosis, your doctor would likely order more blood tests.

If you do not take in enough iron, an iron deficiency anemia may exist. Your levels of hemoglobin and hematocrit would signal if you weren't getting enough iron. This is another potential deficiency in the vegan diet, so it needs to be properly supplemented. To confirm the diagnosis, your doctor will look for signs and symptoms you may have been having and may order a test for serum ferritin and transferrin. If you are iron deficient, your doctor will likely suggest you supplement with iron tablets, which is not a big deal for most people. Some people do experience constipation with iron supplements.

The comprehensive metabolic panel will signal any abnormalities in your electrolytes, your kidney function, your level of hydration, and your protein status. The level of serum creatinine in this panel may indicate that your kidney function (also called your renal function) is insufficient. This is one you should be particularly mindful about because unfortunately, there is more chronic kidney disease in patients than is being detected. A primary reason for this is because many physicians were taught to look primarily at serum creatinine level to detect problems in kidney function. If the serum creatinine appears normal or only slightly elevated, they may not look any further. However, estimated creatinine clearance provides a much more accurate picture of how the kidneys are functioning (also called eGFR or glomerular filtration rate). There are different ways of calculating creatinine clearance, and all have their strengths and weaknesses. Some laboratories are now routinely reporting eGFR (estimated GFR). If your doctor's laboratory is not reporting eGFR, then it is most prudent to ask your doctor what your creatinine clearance would be based on your serum creatinine level. In practice, most clinicians use the Cockgroft-Gault equation. You can find this calculation at http://www.globalrph.com/crcl.htm. Just enter your age, gender, height, weight, and serum creatinine level, and it will calculate your creatinine clearance for you. You can also calculate your own creatinine clearance by working the Cockgroft-Gault equation yourself:

Creatinine Clearance (ml/min) =

(140–age) × weight in kg ÷ (72 × serum creatinine in mg/dl)

If you are female, multiply the above by 0.85 to get your creatinine clearance.

Note: To get weight in kilograms, divide weight in pounds by 2.2. To get weight in pounds, multiply weight in kg by 2.2.

Anything less than 60 ml/min creatinine clearance would be an alert for further evaluation.

The comprehensive metabolic panel will also provide your albumin level, which is a good indicator of nutritional protein status. Protein is made up of building blocks called amino acids. Amino acids are needed for growth to repair body tissue and perform other bodily functions. There are many different types of amino acids, some of which our bodies can manufacture themselves. These are called nonessential amino acids. There are nine amino acids that our bodies cannot manufacture (called essential amino acids) and must get from food sources. Many people are concerned that a vegan diet will not provide enough protein. This is a common misperception. While meat and dairy do provide good sources of protein, vegetable food sources can also provide enough essential amino acids to maintain health. You can prove this to yourself by visiting your doctor and having your blood drawn after following a vegan diet for a couple of months. If your albumin level is within the normal range, then you are getting enough essential amino acids and have an adequate protein status. There is no evidence to the contrary on this subject, so don't be swayed by hucksters who say you need to supplement your amino acid intake with whatever protein supplement they are trying to sell to you.

On your basic metabolic panel, there will be a BUN level (blood urea nitrogen). The BUN to serum creatinine ratio can alert your doctor in a number of ways. A normal BUN:creatinine ratio is 10–20:1 (10 to 20 times higher BUN than creatinine). If the ratio is higher, say 30:1, this may be indicative of dehydration or a more serious condition such as gastrointestinal bleeding. If there are no other symptoms of a more serious health issue, such as black tarry stools or other signs of gastrointestinal bleeding, then it is likely that you are just not drinking enough water. If the ratio is lower than 10:1, say 6:1, it is most likely due to problems with your kidneys; it helps confirm the diagnosis of renal insufficiency if your creatinine clearance was less than 60 ml/minute. The lower ratio can also be indicative of pregnancy, liver disease, or a diet too low in protein. In all cases, if the creatinine level is higher than normal and/or the creatinine clearance calculation is less than 60 ml/min, further investigation is warranted.

Vitamin D level has recently received much attention, mainly because of its association with osteoporosis and heart disease.[3, 4, 5] However, Vitamin D deficiency has also been associated with complications in multiple sclerosis, type 1 diabetes, breast cancer, and others. Although our bodies can make vitamin D with enough sunlight exposure, most of us do not get enough sun exposure to prevent deficiency. And since the risks associated with sun exposure are well known, more sun exposure is not likely to be recommended by your doctor. Vitamin D is not easy to get through food intake; even foods that are fortified with vitamin D often will not provide enough vitamin D to prevent deficiency. Therefore, most of us need to supplement our vitamin D levels by taking a vitamin D supplement. Even if you are already taking a vitamin D supplement, it is a good idea to have your vitamin D level tested to make sure you are getting enough from your supplement.

The thyroid panel is an important test to ensure your thyroid gland is functioning properly. Low thyroid levels can contribute to heart problems, as well as lowering your metabolism (causing you to be overweight) and raising your cholesterol levels, among other problems. High thyroid levels can predispose you to bone fractures and heart arrhythmias (irregular heart beat), among other problems. Problems with your thyroid can be effectively managed, but as with everything else, they first need to be identified. The fasting lipid panel will indicate to you and your doctor if your cholesterol and triglyceride levels are too high, or in the case of HDL cholesterol, too low. LDL cholesterol is the bad cholesterol, responsible for building plaque in your cardiovascular system (called atherosclerosis), which is responsible for putting you at greater risk for heart attacks and strokes, as well as other circulatory problems. The HDL is the good cholesterol that helps to counteract what the LDL is doing. Thus, you want your LDL to be as low as possible, and your HDL to be as high as possible. While lower is better with LDL, with no danger of ever being too low, there are recommended ranges established.[6, 7]

The levels of LDL cholesterol recommended are based on the number of risk factors you have for cardiovascular disease. The recommendations are based on sound evidence derived from analyzing many different scientific research studies. Risk factors include personal and family history, cigarette smoking, hypertension (high blood pressure), diabetes, male gender, advancing age, high saturated fat diet, HDL < 40mg/dl, and obesity. Your consumption of saturated fat, derived from meat products in the diet as well as trans fats, is the largest dietary contributor to your blood level of LDL cholesterol level. This may come as a surprise since most people believe that it is the cholesterol in the diet that causes their blood cholesterol to be elevated, but in fact the greater contributor to blood cholesterol is the amount of saturated fat in the diet. See Table 1 for LDL level recommendations.

Table 1

Risk Category	LDL Goal	Initiate Therapeutic Lifestyle Changes	Consider Drug Therapy
High Risk (10-year risk > 20%)	<100mg/dl	≥ 100mg/dl	≥ 100mg/dl
Moderately High Risk (10-year risk 10%–20%)	<130mg/dl	≥ 130mg/dl	≥ 130mg/dl
Moderate Risk (10-year risk < 10%)	<130mg/dl	≥ 130mg/dl	≥ 160mg/dl
Lower Risk (10-year risk < 10%, and 0–1 risk factors)	<160mg/dl	≥ 160mg/dl	≥ 190mg/dl

Adapted from The National Cholesterol Education Program Report: Implications of Recent Clinical Trials for the National Cholesterol Education Program Adult Treatment Panel III Guidelines. Endorsed by the National Heart, Lung, and Blood Pressure Institute, American College of Cardiology Foundation, and American Heart Association (Circulation, 2004; Vol. 110, pp. 227-239).

Note that your risk category is determined by an equation that takes into account your age, gender, total cholesterol, HDL cholesterol, smoking status, systolic blood pressure, and if you are on medication to control your blood pressure. Your systolic blood pressure is the top number in your blood pressure reading. For example, if your blood pressure is 120/80, your systolic blood pressure is 120. The ten-year risk calculation is available at www.nhlbi.nih.gov/guidelines/cholesterol.

If you are unable to reach the target LDL levels through diet and weight loss, it is likely because you are genetically predisposed to having high LDL levels. Your liver just makes too much of it. In this case, you will need to take medications to reach the target. It is nothing to be ashamed of, and I recommend you don't fight it. It is of high importance to prevent heart attacks and strokes to correct the levels and keep them corrected. The drugs used to lower LDL cholesterol are very safe, with few side effects. Your doctor can monitor for these side effects.

The recommended HDL level is greater than 40 mg/dl, and greater is better, with no apparent limit. Lower levels put you at a higher risk for cardiovascular disease. HDL is not generally affected by your diet but by your genetic propensity and level of exercise. If your HDL level is low, exercise can help raise the level. There are some medications that also raise HDL but not by huge amounts, in general. Drinking red wine in moderation can also help raise the HDL level. Discuss with your physician to get his or her recommendation for a plan to raise your HDL level.

Very Low Density Lipoprotein (VLDL) carries triglyceride throughout the bloodstream, so its level is strongly dependent on the triglyceride level. The target level for fasting triglycerides is less than 150 mg/dl. Higher levels predispose you to a greater risk for cardiovascular complications. High triglycerides can be due to being overweight, having poorly controlled diabetes, drinking too much alcohol, and/or eating too much sugar. They might also show as being high because you were not fasting for the blood test. You should be fasting for eight hours or longer before your lipid panel is drawn. In many cases, triglycerides can be controlled through weight loss, diet correction, and getting diabetes under control. If those efforts do not get them to the target level, there are medications that can help. Again, talk with your physician about his or her recommendations.

Blood sugar levels, both fasting (a minimum of eight hours not having eaten) and two hours after you have eaten (two hours postprandial) can detect diabetes and prediabetes (impaired glucose tolerance [IGT] and impaired fasting glucose [IFG]). Although many physicians still have their patients come in only for a fasting blood sugar, the two-hour postprandial level is oftentimes the first lab value to show that a person has prediabetes.[8] By the time the fasting blood sugar becomes diagnostic, the person may have already progressed to diabetes. Thus, I strongly encourage you to ask your healthcare provider to do both fasting and two hours after eating around 75–100 gm of carbohydrate (equivalent to 20 oz of orange juice, or your doctor may have you drink a sugar solution in the office). See Table 2 for blood glucose levels diagnostic for prediabetes and diabetes. If either of these levels is high, your physician may request an A1c be done. The A1c level reflects average blood glucose over the last two to three months and is also diagnostic for diabetes.

Table 2

Blood Test	Prediabetes	Diabetes
Fasting Blood Sugar	100–125mg/dl	≥ 125 mg/dl
2-Hour Postprandial Blood Sugar	140–199mg/dl	≥ 200mg/dl
A1c	5.7–6.4%	≥ 6.5%

Adapted from the American Diabetes Association's 2012 Position Statement of the Standards of Medical Care in Diabetes (Diabetes Care, Vol. 35, Supplement 1, Jan 2012, pp.S11-S63).

Remember that if you have prediabetes, there is hope in preventing type 2 diabetes.

The C-reactive protein (CRP) level gives an indication of the level of inflammatory response going on inside your body[9], and if chronically elevated, it can add to the predictive value of total and HDL cholesterol in determining the risk of heart attacks and strokes in both men and women.[10,11] While there are also other biomarkers of inflammation, they are not yet routinely tested in practice. Be aware that recent trauma and infection can also cause the CRP level to become elevated. Thus, if your level is elevated, your doctor may wish to get a repeat blood sample at a later date to confirm the level is chronically elevated. There are a few means by which your CRP can be lowered. Following a vegan diet can actually reduce the level of CRP to the same extent as taking a statin![12,13] Increasing physical activity can lower CRP level[14], as can the statins used to lower LDL levels.[15] You may wish to discuss with your physician your desire to try the 95% vegan diet approach before starting medication. The key is that if you attempt to reduce the level with the 95% vegan diet approach, you need to recheck your CRP in about three months to ensure it has gotten your CRP level into the acceptable range. If not, it is time to seriously consider taking the statin.

Liver function tests (LFTs) can help detect numerous abnormalities which can be due to a multitude of causes including liver damage from alcohol abuse, taking certain medications, viral and autoimmune hepatitis, gastrointestinal infection, and bile duct obstruction.[16]

To conclude in a nutshell, unless you have some rare condition that dictates otherwise (and you would likely know this), the steps outlined here for you represent an excellent start to partner with your physician and monitor your own health and nutritional status. Since science is ever evolving, other measurements may make their way to the forefront for testing in your healthcare provider's office. If you stay current on scientifically validated instruments to test your health, you will remain effective at managing your own health with your healthcare provider.

DIRECTIONS

If you have had recent blood work drawn at your doctor's office, request that a copy of your results be sent to you. Compare the results to the recommendations in this section. Record results in the table provided below. If you have not had a recent physical, schedule one with your physician now. Bring this workbook with you to your appointment in order to discuss what you would like to have done and any other recommendations your physician may have for you. Be sure to ask your physician to have the results of your blood work and urinalysis sent to you, so that you can record your results here. If any levels concern you that have not already been discussed with your doctor, notify his or her office that you need to speak with your doctor. Ask for his or her recommendations, including when you should schedule your next appointment for follow-up. Record his or her recommendations in the lab value table below so that you can remind yourself as well as follow-up with her at your next appointment. Keeping up with your own health is a great way to have more productive discussions with your physician during your appointments.

Remember, you can't fix something if you don't know it is broken. I implore you not to stick your head in the sand regarding your health; many health problems can be avoided or minimized through routine health checkups. Just feeling okay doesn't mean you are okay!

Lab Test	Date	Result	Date	Result
Blood Pressure:				
Systolic				
Diastolic				
Physician's Recommendation:				
Comprehensive Metabolic Panel				
All electrolytes within normal limits? (Y/N)				
If abnormal, why?				
Physician's Recommendation:				
BUN (mg/dl)				
Serum Creatinine (mg/dl)				
BUN:Creatinine Ratio Normal? (Y/N)				
If abnormal, why?				
Creatinine Clearance or eGFR (ml/min)				
If creatinine clearance less than 60 ml/min, what is physician's recommendation?				
Albumin level normal?				
If not, why?				
Physician's Recommendation:				
CBC				
Hemoglobin				
Hematocrit				
White count normal?(Y/N)				
Signs of macrocytic anemia? (Y/N)				
Physician's Recommendation:				
Blood Glucose				
Fasting				
2 hours postprandial (after eating)				
A1c				
Other				
Physician's Recommendation:				
Lipid Panel				
LDL(mg/dl)				
HDL(mg/dl)				
VLDL(mg/dl)				
Triglycerides(mg/dl)				
Physician's Recommendation:				
Thyroid Panel Results - Normal, Abnormal				
Physician's Recommendation:				
Vitamin D Level - Low, Normal, High				
Physician's Recommendation:				

THE 95% VEGAN DIET WORKBOOK

Lab Test	Date	Result	Date	Result
Blood Pressure:				
Systolic				
Diastolic				
Physician's Recommendation:				
Comprehensive Metabolic Panel				
All electrolytes within normal limits? (Y/N)				
If abnormal, why?				
Physician's Recommendation:				
BUN (mg/dl)				
Serum Creatinine (mg/dl)				
BUN:Creatinine Ratio Normal? (Y/N)				
If abnormal, why?				
Creatinine Clearance or eGFR (ml/min)				
If creatinine clearance less than 60 ml/min, what is physician's recommendation?				
Albumin level normal?				
If not, why?				
Physician's Recommendation:				
CBC				
Hemoglobin				
Hematocrit				
White count normal?(Y/N)				
Signs of macrocytic anemia? (Y/N)				
Physician's Recommendation:				
Blood Glucose				
Fasting				
2 hours postprandial (after eating)				
A1c				
Other				
Physician's Recommendation:				
Lipid Panel				
LDL(mg/dl)				
HDL(mg/dl)				
VLDL(mg/dl)				
Triglycerides(mg/dl)				
Physician's Recommendation:				
Thyroid Panel Results - Normal, Abnormal				
Physician's Recommendation:				
Vitamin D Level - Low, Normal, High				
Physician's Recommendation:				

Lab Test	Date	Result	Date	Result
Blood Pressure:				
Systolic				
Diastolic				
Physician's Recommendation:				
Comprehensive Metabolic Panel				
All electrolytes within normal limits? (Y/N)				
If abnormal, why?				
Physician's Recommendation:				
BUN (mg/dl)				
Serum Creatinine (mg/dl)				
BUN:Creatinine Ratio Normal? (Y/N)				
If abnormal, why?				
Creatinine Clearance or eGFR (ml/min)				
If creatinine clearance less than 60 ml/min, what is physician's recommendation?				
Albumin level normal?				
If not, why?				
Physician's Recommendation:				
CBC				
Hemoglobin				
Hematocrit				
White count normal?(Y/N)				
Signs of macrocytic anemia? (Y/N)				
Physician's Recommendation:				
Blood Glucose				
Fasting				
2 hours postprandial (after eating)				
A1c				
Other				
Physician's Recommendation:				
Lipid Panel				
LDL(mg/dl)				
HDL(mg/dl)				
VLDL(mg/dl)				
Triglycerides(mg/dl)				
Physician's Recommendation:				
Thyroid Panel Results - Normal, Abnormal				
Physician's Recommendation:				
Vitamin D Level - Low, Normal, High				
Physician's Recommendation:				

THE 95% VEGAN DIET WORKBOOK

Lab Test	Date	Result	Date	Result
Blood Pressure:				
Systolic				
Diastolic				
Physician's Recommendation:				
Comprehensive Metabolic Panel				
All electrolytes within normal limits? (Y/N)				
If abnormal, why?				
Physician's Recommendation:				
BUN (mg/dl)				
Serum Creatinine (mg/dl)				
BUN:Creatinine Ratio Normal? (Y/N)				
If abnormal, why?				
Creatinine Clearance or eGFR (ml/min)				
If creatinine clearance less than 60 ml/min, what is physician's recommendation?				
Albumin level normal?				
If not, why?				
Physician's Recommendation:				
CBC				
Hemoglobin				
Hematocrit				
White count normal?(Y/N)				
Signs of macrocytic anemia? (Y/N)				
Physician's Recommendation:				
Blood Glucose				
Fasting				
2 hours postprandial (after eating)				
A1c				
Other				
Physician's Recommendation:				
Lipid Panel				
LDL(mg/dl)				
HDL(mg/dl)				
VLDL(mg/dl)				
Triglycerides(mg/dl)				
Physician's Recommendation:				
Thyroid Panel Results - Normal, Abnormal				
Physician's Recommendation:				
Vitamin D Level - Low, Normal, High				
Physician's Recommendation:				

Lab Test	Date	Result	Date	Result
Blood Pressure:				
Systolic				
Diastolic				
Physician's Recommendation:				
Comprehensive Metabolic Panel				
All electrolytes within normal limits? (Y/N)				
If abnormal, why?				
Physician's Recommendation:				
BUN (mg/dl)				
Serum Creatinine (mg/dl)				
BUN:Creatinine Ratio Normal? (Y/N)				
If abnormal, why?				
Creatinine Clearance or eGFR (ml/min)				
If creatinine clearance less than 60 ml/min, what is physician's recommendation?				
Albumin level normal?				
If not, why?				
Physician's Recommendation:				
CBC				
Hemoglobin				
Hematocrit				
White count normal?(Y/N)				
Signs of macrocytic anemia? (Y/N)				
Physician's Recommendation:				
Blood Glucose				
Fasting				
2 hours postprandial (after eating)				
A1c				
Other				
Physician's Recommendation:				
Lipid Panel				
LDL(mg/dl)				
HDL(mg/dl)				
VLDL(mg/dl)				
Triglycerides(mg/dl)				
Physician's Recommendation:				
Thyroid Panel Results - Normal, Abnormal				
Physician's Recommendation:				
Vitamin D Level - Low, Normal, High				
Physician's Recommendation:				

THE 95% VEGAN DIET WORKBOOK

Lab Test	Date	Result	Date	Result
Blood Pressure:				
Systolic				
Diastolic				
Physician's Recommendation:				
Comprehensive Metabolic Panel				
All electrolytes within normal limits? (Y/N)				
If abnormal, why?				
Physician's Recommendation:				
BUN (mg/dl)				
Serum Creatinine (mg/dl)				
BUN:Creatinine Ratio Normal? (Y/N)				
If abnormal, why?				
Creatinine Clearance or eGFR (ml/min)				
If creatinine clearance less than 60 ml/min, what is physician's recommendation?				
Albumin level normal?				
If not, why?				
Physician's Recommendation:				
CBC				
Hemoglobin				
Hematocrit				
White count normal?(Y/N)				
Signs of macrocytic anemia? (Y/N)				
Physician's Recommendation:				
Blood Glucose				
Fasting				
2 hours postprandial (after eating)				
A1c				
Other				
Physician's Recommendation:				
Lipid Panel				
LDL(mg/dl)				
HDL(mg/dl)				
VLDL(mg/dl)				
Triglycerides(mg/dl)				
Physician's Recommendation:				
Thyroid Panel Results - Normal, Abnormal				
Physician's Recommendation:				
Vitamin D Level - Low, Normal, High				
Physician's Recommendation:				

Lab Test	Date	Result	Date	Result
Blood Pressure:				
Systolic				
Diastolic				
Physician's Recommendation:				
Comprehensive Metabolic Panel				
All electrolytes within normal limits? (Y/N)				
If abnormal, why?				
Physician's Recommendation:				
BUN (mg/dl)				
Serum Creatinine (mg/dl)				
BUN:Creatinine Ratio Normal? (Y/N)				
If abnormal, why?				
Creatinine Clearance or eGFR (ml/min)				
If creatinine clearance less than 60 ml/min, what is physician's recommendation?				
Albumin level normal?				
If not, why?				
Physician's Recommendation:				
CBC				
Hemoglobin				
Hematocrit				
White count normal?(Y/N)				
Signs of macrocytic anemia? (Y/N)				
Physician's Recommendation:				
Blood Glucose				
Fasting				
2 hours postprandial (after eating)				
A1c				
Other				
Physician's Recommendation:				
Lipid Panel				
LDL(mg/dl)				
HDL(mg/dl)				
VLDL(mg/dl)				
Triglycerides(mg/dl)				
Physician's Recommendation:				
Thyroid Panel Results - Normal, Abnormal				
Physician's Recommendation:				
Vitamin D Level - Low, Normal, High				
Physician's Recommendation:				

THE 95% VEGAN DIET WORKBOOK

Lab Test	Date	Result	Date	Result
Blood Pressure:				
Systolic				
Diastolic				
Physician's Recommendation:				
Comprehensive Metabolic Panel				
All electrolytes within normal limits? (Y/N)				
If abnormal, why?				
Physician's Recommendation:				
BUN (mg/dl)				
Serum Creatinine (mg/dl)				
BUN:Creatinine Ratio Normal? (Y/N)				
If abnormal, why?				
Creatinine Clearance or eGFR (ml/min)				
If creatinine clearance less than 60 ml/min, what is physician's recommendation?				
Albumin level normal?				
If not, why?				
Physician's Recommendation:				
CBC				
Hemoglobin				
Hematocrit				
White count normal?(Y/N)				
Signs of macrocytic anemia? (Y/N)				
Physician's Recommendation:				
Blood Glucose				
Fasting				
2 hours postprandial (after eating)				
A1c				
Other				
Physician's Recommendation:				
Lipid Panel				
LDL(mg/dl)				
HDL(mg/dl)				
VLDL(mg/dl)				
Triglycerides(mg/dl)				
Physician's Recommendation:				
Thyroid Panel Results - Normal, Abnormal				
Physician's Recommendation:				
Vitamin D Level - Low, Normal, High				
Physician's Recommendation:				

Lab Test	Date	Result	Date	Result
Blood Pressure:				
Systolic				
Diastolic				
Physician's Recommendation:				
Comprehensive Metabolic Panel				
All electrolytes within normal limits? (Y/N)				
If abnormal, why?				
Physician's Recommendation:				
BUN (mg/dl)				
Serum Creatinine (mg/dl)				
BUN:Creatinine Ratio Normal? (Y/N)				
If abnormal, why?				
Creatinine Clearance or eGFR (ml/min)				
If creatinine clearance less than 60 ml/min, what is physician's recommendation?				
Albumin level normal?				
If not, why?				
Physician's Recommendation:				
CBC				
Hemoglobin				
Hematocrit				
White count normal?(Y/N)				
Signs of macrocytic anemia? (Y/N)				
Physician's Recommendation:				
Blood Glucose				
Fasting				
2 hours postprandial (after eating)				
A1c				
Other				
Physician's Recommendation:				
Lipid Panel				
LDL(mg/dl)				
HDL(mg/dl)				
VLDL(mg/dl)				
Triglycerides(mg/dl)				
Physician's Recommendation:				
Thyroid Panel Results - Normal, Abnormal				
Physician's Recommendation:				
Vitamin D Level - Low, Normal, High				
Physician's Recommendation:				

THE 95% VEGAN DIET WORKBOOK

Lab Test	Date	Result	Date	Result
Blood Pressure:				
Systolic				
Diastolic				
Physician's Recommendation:				
Comprehensive Metabolic Panel				
All electrolytes within normal limits? (Y/N)				
If abnormal, why?				
Physician's Recommendation:				
BUN (mg/dl)				
Serum Creatinine (mg/dl)				
BUN:Creatinine Ratio Normal? (Y/N)				
If abnormal, why?				
Creatinine Clearance or eGFR (ml/min)				
If creatinine clearance less than 60 ml/min, what is physician's recommendation?				
Albumin level normal?				
If not, why?				
Physician's Recommendation:				
CBC				
Hemoglobin				
Hematocrit				
White count normal?(Y/N)				
Signs of macrocytic anemia? (Y/N)				
Physician's Recommendation:				
Blood Glucose				
Fasting				
2 hours postprandial (after eating)				
A1c				
Other				
Physician's Recommendation:				
Lipid Panel				
LDL(mg/dl)				
HDL(mg/dl)				
VLDL(mg/dl)				
Triglycerides(mg/dl)				
Physician's Recommendation:				
Thyroid Panel Results - Normal, Abnormal				
Physician's Recommendation:				
Vitamin D Level - Low, Normal, High				
Physician's Recommendation:				

THE MACRONUTRIENTS, WATER, FIBER, AND ORGANIC

In this chapter, we will begin to get more specific about taking control of your dietary intake. Keep in mind that, although I will provide specific guidelines, if you are eating a vegan diet with a wide array or food choices, adding very little fat, you will be getting what your body needs in terms of carbohydrate and protein.

CARBOHYDRATE

In this section, you can keep up with the glycemic load of the carbohydrate content of your diet. Glycemic load is a calculation in which the glycemic index is multiplied by the total number of carbs, minus the grams of fiber, and divided by 100.[1]

$$\text{glycemic load} = \frac{\text{glycemic index} \times \text{total available carbs (total grams carb–fiber)}}{100}$$

A score of 1–10 is considered to be a low glycemic load, 11–19 is a medium load, and 20 or higher is considered a high glycemic load.

	A	B	C	D	E	F	G	H
	Food	Approximate Portion Size	Total Carb	Dietary Fiber	Available Carb (C - D)	Glycemic Index	Glycemic Load (E X F ÷100)	Low, Medium or High Glycemic Load?*
EXAMPLES								
Hummus	1/4 cup	8g	2g	6g	6	0.36	Low
Maple and brown sugar instant oatmeal	1 packet	33g	3g	30g	83	24.9	High
Pitted prunes	2 pitted	12g	1.5g	10.5g	29	3	Low
* 1-10 = low glycemic load, 11-19 = medium, 20 or greater - high glycemic load								

THE 95% VEGAN DIET WORKBOOK

A	B	C	D	E	F	G	H
Food	Approximate Portion Size	Total Carb	Dietary Fiber	Available Carb (C - D)	Glycemic Index	Glycemic Load (E X F ÷100)	Low, Medium or High Glycemic Load?*

FAT

First, calculate the total *maximum* number of fat grams you should have in one day.

A	B	C	D
Desired Weight in Pounds*	Multiply desired weight in pounds by 15 for a quick approximation of calories per day to maintain that weight (Column A X 15)	Multiply total calories by 0.3 (30%) to get total maximum calories from all fat sources Column B X 0.3)	Divide total calories by 9 to get grams per day of maximum total fat grams per day
EXAMPLE:			
135	2025	607.5	67.5

Calculate the healthy fat intake recommendation specific to you.

GUIDELINES FOR FAT INTAKE SPECIFIC TO YOU					
A	B	C	D	E	F
Desired Weight in Pounds*	Multiply desired weight in pounds by 15 for a quick approximation of calories per day to maintain that weight (Column A X 15)	Multiply total calories by 1.6% (0.016) to get calories from Omega-3's (Column B X 0.016)	Divide total calories by 9 to get grams per day of Omega-3's (Column C/9)	Multiply total calories by 5% (0.050)) to get calories from Omega-6's (Column B X 0.050)	Divide by 9 to get grams per day of Omega-6's(Column F/9)
EXAMPLE:					
135	2025	32.4	3.6	101	11

*Refer back to the previous HOMEWORK assignment in which you identified the weight you need to be in order to have a BMI of less than 25. If BMI did not apply to you, then enter the weight you wish to maintain long-term.

PROTEIN

Absolute protein requirements are most dependent on weight.[2] For women, 0.85gm/kg (0.39 gm/lb) body weight is a good estimate. For men, around 1 gm/kg (0.45gm/lb) body weight is a good estimate.[3] For women, as they get older, more protein may be needed to preserve muscle mass, ensure adequate calcium absorption, and help minimize bone loss—1gm/kg (0.45gm/lb) body weight.[4,5,6] Use the following table to calculate the appropriate amount of daily protein in your diet:

A	B	C	D	E	F
Gender	Age	Weight in Pounds	Divide Column C by 2.2 to get weight in kg	GM/KG Protein Required (1gm for men, 0.85gm for women under 65, and 1gm for women over 65)	Multiply Column D X Column E to get grams of protein required per Day
Male	18 and above			1.00	
Women	<65 years			0.85	
Women	≥ 65 years			1.00	
EXAMPLES					
Male	48	180	81.8	1.00	82
Female	36	135	61.4	0.85	52
Older Female	70	128	58.2	1.00	58

As you can see from the examples, a man weighing 180 pounds requires 82 grams of protein per day, a woman less than sixty-five years of age who weighs 135 pounds requires 52 grams of protein per day, and a woman over the age of sixty-five who weighs 128 pounds likely requires 58 grams of protein per day.

The average Western diet contains two to three times as much protein as is needed. It's no surprise that Americans are a standout population in terms of obesity and cardiovascular disease! Along with the excessive protein, we are getting far too much fat. By switching to vegetable sources for your protein needs, it is possible to cut out pretty much all fat. For example, legumes (beans and peas) and tofu contain very little fat. On the other hand, nuts and seeds contain quite a bit of fat. And just because nuts and seeds contain "good fat," if you have a high LDL, no fat is a good fat for you other than the bare essentials we discussed above. You would not be helping yourself to consume more nuts with the idea that they are "heart healthy."

Now comes the question about the *quality* of protein in the vegan diet. Protein derived from animal sources has been traditionally called *high biological value* or *complete protein* because it contains all of the essential amino acids (the ones your body cannot manufacture). If you are getting all of your protein from plant sources, unless you get it all from isolated soy protein (you won't) or nutritional yeast flakes,* you will get more of certain essential amino acids from beans and legumes and more of other essential amino acids from grains. And although it is still widely believed that because of the lower digestibility of plant foods versus animal sources means vegans must eat more protein, studies show that there is not a significant difference in protein requirements based on the source of the protein intake.[7] This means that the amount you calculated for yourself above does

---

* Nutritional yeast flakes are used in many vegan recipes. Two tablespoons provides a whopping eight grams of complete protein.

not need to be adjusted up because you will be getting the majority, if not all, of your protein needs from plant sources.

Beans and legumes are particularly high in lysine, while grains provide more methionine. Together, they provide complete protein. However, because your diet will be relatively high in grains (whole grain breads, rice. and pasta) already, you do not generally need to worry about whether you are getting enough methionine. Note also that all of the other essential amino acids pretty much balance out over your entire dietary intake.

Your attention should be more attuned to whether you are getting enough lysine than getting enough methionine. In addition to eating beans and legumes, you will get lysine through using soy milk, green leafy vegetables, potatoes (both sweet and white), and squash. Other vegetables also contain lysine, just in lesser quantities. This is why you always hear that with a varied diet, you can meet your nutritional needs.

Another theory we need to discuss is the one that tells us we must eat complementary proteins at the same time in order for the body to use your protein intake properly. This is not the case. Because our muscles contain a pool of free amino acids for the body to use, particularly lysine, you do not have to ensure you eat complementary proteins within the same meal or even the same time span. In fact, as long as you average a sufficient intake of essential amino acids over several days, you should be fine.[8]

WATER

· ·

See http://water.epa.gov/drink/standardsriskmanagement.cfm for the Environmental Protection Agency's drinking water standards. Your city can set its own standards for water quality, which can be more stringent than the EPA guidelines but never less stringent than EPA guidelines. If your water supply comes from a well, you are pretty much on your own to ensure your water is safe to drink and bathe in.

There are all sorts of potential water contaminants out there, including pesticides, disinfectants, radioactive substances, and dangerous byproducts of industry, such as chromium VI (also called hexavalent chromium). The good news is that the EPA and cities are on top of water testing and have maximum levels allowed where there is science to support maximum safe levels. The bad news is that science is ever evolving, and what was considered safe ten years ago, may not be considered safe today. Thus, we may have been exposed to toxic levels of various chemicals through no fault of the EPA—the science may just not have been there at the time. The other bad news is that if there is a water main break, your water can become easily contaminated to the point where it is considered not potable (not safe to drink) or even safe to bathe in. Again, if you are on well water, it is up to you to ensure your water is safe. Let's discuss this further.

NSF International (National Sanitation Foundation), a nonprofit, nongovernmental organization, is the leading global provider of safety standards for concerned citizens worldwide. It certifies various products through testing and retesting to meet their set standards, including drinking water purification systems. You can find the standards for drinking water at http://www.nsf.org/business/drinking_water_treatment/standards.asp. There are three standards to be aware of, in terms of removing contaminants from drinking water:

1. NSF 42 – A filtration system meeting this standard improves the aesthetics of the water. It reduces odors, removes particulates, and reduces chlorine. Many refrigerators with water dispensers have this level of filter.

2. NSF 53 – A filtration system meeting this standard reduces specific contaminants that can impact health, such as lead, volatile organic chemicals (VOCs) such as benzene, and microorganisms such as cryptosporidium and giardia. It filters out chemicals that have a molecular weight or atomic mass roughly of one hundred or more. The terms *molecular weight* and

45

atomic mass refer to the size of the contaminant. Lead has an atomic mass of around 207, so a product that meets NSF 53 would filter it out.

3. NSF 58 – A filtration system meeting this standard cleans water through a reverse osmosis system, which further reduces contamination from additional potential poisons such as trivalent and hexavalent chromium (chromium III and chromium VI respectively), nitrates, and other dissolved solvents. It also removes fluoride and other minerals. Essentially, it removes smaller molecules than filters satisfying NSF 53, less than 100 molecular weight or atomic mass. The atomic mass of hexavalent chromium VI is 43, much smaller than lead. Fluoride's atomic mass is around 18.

The NSF standard to cover softening hard water, particularly for those on well water is NSF 44. Other NSF standards cover different methods of purifying drinking water (mostly for public waterworks) and filter systems for shower and bath.

There are many good filtration systems on the market that meet NSF 42 and 53 standards. You can choose whether you would want an above-the-counter model, which attaches directly to your sink faucet or an under-the-counter system, in which another hole is drilled for an additional faucet. If you already have a filtration system or are using a product that is a pitcher with a filtration system, you may want to do a little digging to determine which NSF standards the product meets. Most of the pitcher type models only cover NSF 42.

Reverse osmosis systems satisfying NSF 58 are also available for residential use. Most of them require an under-the-counter configuration, in which you would gain an additional faucet, but above the counter models are now emerging. The price of these systems has come down tremendously very recently so are affordable for much of the population. If you are handy as a plumber, you can probably install the system without any help.

SUGGESTED STEPS TO HELP ENSURE YOUR DRINKING WATER IS SAFE

1. Whether you are on city or well water, get the list of the national drinking water standards from http://water.epa.gov/drink/contaminants/upload/mcl-2.pdf.

2. If you are on city water, you can go to http://cfpub.epa.gov/safewater/ccr/index.cfm? OpenView to view the most recent water testing report for your water provider. Compare it to the drinking water standards.

3. If you are on well water and do not routinely monitor your water supply, you can request an agent test a sample for known poisons (on the list you obtained from step 1). Go to http://www.cdc.gov/healthywater/drinking/private/wells/faq.html to find out how to get your water tested. As you will see, the EPA clearly states that you are responsible for the safety of your own well water. Click on all of the applicable links to thoroughly learn what

you do not yet know. You can either have your water tested for you through a company (or sending in a sample to a laboratory) or you can purchase a testing kit and do it yourself. Please be aware that many at-home testing kits may only test for hardness, chlorine, and microorganisms. You want more thorough testing than that. Just be sure you know what you are getting before you invest.

4. Based on what you have learned about your drinking water, decide whether or not you believe you need a filtration or reverse osmosis system. The decision is entirely up to you.

5. Once you decide if you need a system and desired NSF standards it will need to meet, you can either shop locally for it or Google for "water purification systems." You will find a multitude of choices out there.

FIBER

Unless otherwise directed, your intake of fiber daily should be 25 grams or more or women and 38 grams or more for men.[9] You can easily find fiber content of various foods at www.calorieking.com. You can use any other resource at your disposal instead, if you wish.

In order to help you keep up with your daily fiber intake, record content of various foods from your 95% Vegan diet in the table below.

Food	Quantity	Fiber Content in Gms

Food	Quantity	Fiber Content in Gms

ORGANIC OR NOT?

. . . .

Go to http://www.ewg.org/foodnews/summary/, and find the *Dirty Dozen*™ and *Clean 15*™. The Dirty Dozen are the foods that should always be purchased organic, if at all possible. The Clean 15 are the foods containing the lowest amount of pesticides and herbicides. Record the current lists here for your reference:

DIRTY DOZEN™

CLEAN 15™

READING LABELS FOR VEGANISM

Reading labels to ensure a product is 100% vegan is an important step to ensure you stay 95% vegan. If you are allowing yourself to eat one meat/dairy containing meal per week, then it is important that you ensure the rest of your week is 100 percent vegan to achieve 95 percent for that week overall. However, you may find that some of the things you have really enjoyed were already vegan.

List here your favorite commercially prepared foods that you have discovered are vegan:

VEGAN FRUGAL FUN BY THE SEASON

In this section, you have the opportunity to keep track of vegan recipes you have made by the season and for each holiday for five years or more. This way, you can keep up with what you and your family enjoyed, and build upon your success from year to year!

SPRING [MARCH 21-JUNE 20]

SPRING'S SEASONAL FRUITS AND VEGETABLES

apples	artichokes	asparagus
avocados	broccoli	Brussels sprouts
cabbage	cauliflower	celery
chard	cherries	collards
dates	fava beans	fennel
grapefruit	jicama	kale
kumquats	leeks	lemons
lettuce	limes	Mandarin oranges
mushrooms	oranges	parsnips
parsnips	pomelos	potatoes
radishes	scallions	shallots
strawberries	tangerines	turnips

55

Year	Favorite Recipes	Recipe Location	Ingredients Needed
	1.		
	2.		
	3.		
	4.		
	5.		
	6.		
	7.		
	8.		
	9.		
	10.		
	1.		
	2.		
	3.		
	4.		
	5.		
	6.		
	7.		
	8.		
	9.		
	10.		
	1.		
	2.		
	3.		
	4.		
	5.		
	6.		
	7.		
	8.		
	9.		
	10.		

THE 95% VEGAN DIET WORKBOOK

Year	Favorite Recipes	Recipe Location	Ingredients Needed
_____	1. _____	_____	_____
	2. _____	_____	_____
	3. _____	_____	_____
	4. _____	_____	_____
	5. _____	_____	_____
	6. _____	_____	_____
	7. _____	_____	_____
	8. _____	_____	_____
	9. _____	_____	_____
	10. _____	_____	_____
_____	1. _____	_____	_____
	2. _____	_____	_____
	3. _____	_____	_____
	4. _____	_____	_____
	5. _____	_____	_____
	6. _____	_____	_____
	7. _____	_____	_____
	8. _____	_____	_____
	9. _____	_____	_____
	10. _____	_____	_____

ST. PATRICK'S DAY

Year	Recipes	Recipe Location	Grocery List
	1.		
	2.		
	3.		
	4.		
	5.		
	6.		
	7.		
	8.		
	9.		
	10.		
	1.		
	2.		
	3.		
	4.		
	5.		
	6.		
	7.		
	8.		
	9.		
	10.		
	1.		
	2.		
	3.		
	4.		
	5.		
	6.		
	7.		
	8.		
	9.		
	10.		

THE 95% VEGAN DIET WORKBOOK

ST. PATRICK'S DAY

Year	Recipes	Recipe Location	Grocery List
____	1. _____	_____	_____
	2. _____	_____	_____
	3. _____	_____	_____
	4. _____	_____	_____
	5. _____	_____	_____
	6. _____	_____	_____
	7. _____	_____	_____
	8. _____	_____	_____
	9. _____	_____	_____
	10. _____	_____	_____
____	1. _____	_____	_____
	2. _____	_____	_____
	3. _____	_____	_____
	4. _____	_____	_____
	5. _____	_____	_____
	6. _____	_____	_____
	7. _____	_____	_____
	8. _____	_____	_____
	9. _____	_____	_____
	10. _____	_____	_____

EARTH DAY

Year	Recipes	Recipe Location	Grocery List
_____	1. _____ 2. _____ 3. _____ 4. _____ 5. _____ 6. _____ 7. _____ 8. _____ 9. _____ 10. _____	_____ _____ _____ _____ _____ _____ _____ _____ _____ _____	_____ _____ _____ _____ _____ _____ _____ _____ _____ _____
_____	1. _____ 2. _____ 3. _____ 4. _____ 5. _____ 6. _____ 7. _____ 8. _____ 9. _____ 10. _____	_____ _____ _____ _____ _____ _____ _____ _____ _____ _____	_____ _____ _____ _____ _____ _____ _____ _____ _____ _____
_____	1. _____ 2. _____ 3. _____ 4. _____ 5. _____ 6. _____ 7. _____ 8. _____ 9. _____ 10. _____	_____ _____ _____ _____ _____ _____ _____ _____ _____ _____	_____ _____ _____ _____ _____ _____ _____ _____ _____ _____

EARTH DAY

Year	Recipes	Recipe Location	Grocery List
_____	1. _____	_____	_____
	2. _____	_____	_____
	3. _____	_____	_____
	4. _____	_____	_____
	5. _____	_____	_____
	6. _____	_____	_____
	7. _____	_____	_____
	8. _____	_____	_____
	9. _____	_____	_____
	10. _____	_____	_____
_____	1. _____	_____	_____
	2. _____	_____	_____
	3. _____	_____	_____
	4. _____	_____	_____
	5. _____	_____	_____
	6. _____	_____	_____
	7. _____	_____	_____
	8. _____	_____	_____
	9. _____	_____	_____
	10. _____	_____	_____

EASTER

Year	Recipes	Recipe Location	Grocery List
	1.		
	2.		
	3.		
	4.		
	5.		
	6.		
	7.		
	8.		
	9.		
	10.		
	1.		
	2.		
	3.		
	4.		
	5.		
	6.		
	7.		
	8.		
	9.		
	10.		
	1.		
	2.		
	3.		
	4.		
	5.		
	6.		
	7.		
	8.		
	9.		
	10.		

THE 95% VEGAN DIET WORKBOOK

EASTER

Year	Recipes	Recipe Location	Grocery List
_____	1. _____ 2. _____ 3. _____ 4. _____ 5. _____ 6. _____ 7. _____ 8. _____ 9. _____ 10. _____		
_____	1. _____ 2. _____ 3. _____ 4. _____ 5. _____ 6. _____ 7. _____ 8. _____ 9. _____ 10. _____		

CINCO DE MAYO

Year	Recipes	Recipe Location	Grocery List
	1.		
	2.		
	3.		
	4.		
	5.		
	6.		
	7.		
	8.		
	9.		
	10.		
	1.		
	2.		
	3.		
	4.		
	5.		
	6.		
	7.		
	8.		
	9.		
	10.		
	1.		
	2.		
	3.		
	4.		
	5.		
	6.		
	7.		
	8.		
	9.		
	10.		

THE 95% VEGAN DIET WORKBOOK

CINCO DE MAYO

Year	Recipes	Recipe Location	Grocery List
_____	1. _____	_____	_____
	2. _____	_____	_____
	3. _____	_____	_____
	4. _____	_____	_____
	5. _____	_____	_____
	6. _____	_____	_____
	7. _____	_____	_____
	8. _____	_____	_____
	9. _____	_____	_____
	10. _____	_____	_____
_____	1. _____	_____	_____
	2. _____	_____	_____
	3. _____	_____	_____
	4. _____	_____	_____
	5. _____	_____	_____
	6. _____	_____	_____
	7. _____	_____	_____
	8. _____	_____	_____
	9. _____	_____	_____
	10. _____	_____	_____

SUMMER [JUNE 21–SEPTEMBER 21]

SEASONAL FRUITS AND VEGETABLES

apricots	arugula	avocados
beets	blackberries	blueberries
boysenberries	broccoli	cabbage
cactus pears	carrots	cauliflower
celery	cherries	corn
cucumbers	dates	eggplant
figs	ginger	grapes
green beans	lemons	lettuce
melons	mulberries	nectarines
okra	olives	onions
oranges	peaches	peanuts
peas	peppers	plums
pluots	raspberries	rhubarb
spinach	strawberries	tayberries
tomatoes		

Year	Favorite Recipes	Recipe Location	Ingredients Needed
_____	1. _____ 2. _____ 3. _____ 4. _____ 5. _____ 6. _____ 7. _____ 8. _____ 9. _____ 10. _____		
_____	1. _____ 2. _____ 3. _____ 4. _____ 5. _____ 6. _____ 7. _____ 8. _____ 9. _____ 10. _____		
_____	1. _____ 2. _____ 3. _____ 4. _____ 5. _____ 6. _____ 7. _____ 8. _____ 9. _____ 10. _____		

THE 95% VEGAN DIET WORKBOOK

Year	Favorite Recipes	Recipe Location	Ingredients Needed
_____	1. _____	_____	_____
	2. _____	_____	_____
	3. _____	_____	_____
	4. _____	_____	_____
	5. _____	_____	_____
	6. _____	_____	_____
	7. _____	_____	_____
	8. _____	_____	_____
	9. _____	_____	_____
	10. _____	_____	_____
_____	1. _____	_____	_____
	2. _____	_____	_____
	3. _____	_____	_____
	4. _____	_____	_____
	5. _____	_____	_____
	6. _____	_____	_____
	7. _____	_____	_____
	8. _____	_____	_____
	9. _____	_____	_____
	10. _____	_____	_____

JULY FOURTH

Year	Favorite Recipes	Recipe Location	Ingredients Needed
_____	1. _____ 2. _____ 3. _____ 4. _____ 5. _____ 6. _____ 7. _____ 8. _____ 9. _____ 10. _____		
_____	1. _____ 2. _____ 3. _____ 4. _____ 5. _____ 6. _____ 7. _____ 8. _____ 9. _____ 10. _____		
_____	1. _____ 2. _____ 3. _____ 4. _____ 5. _____ 6. _____ 7. _____ 8. _____ 9. _____ 10. _____		

JULY FOURTH

Year	Favorite Recipes	Recipe Location	Ingredients Needed
	1.		
	2.		
	3.		
	4.		
	5.		
	6.		
	7.		
	8.		
	9.		
	10.		
	1.		
	2.		
	3.		
	4.		
	5.		
	6.		
	7.		
	8.		
	9.		
	10.		

THE FEAST OF MOTHER CABRINI [AUG 24-SEPT 3]

Year	Favorite Recipes	Recipe Location	Ingredients Needed
	1.		
	2.		
	3.		
	4.		
	5.		
	6.		
	7.		
	8.		
	9.		
	10.		
	1.		
	2.		
	3.		
	4.		
	5.		
	6.		
	7.		
	8.		
	9.		
	10.		
	1.		
	2.		
	3.		
	4.		
	5.		
	6.		
	7.		
	8.		
	9.		
	10.		

THE FEAST OF MOTHER CABRINI [AUG 24-SEPT 3]

Year	Favorite Recipes	Recipe Location	Ingredients Needed
_____	1. _____ 2. _____ 3. _____ 4. _____ 5. _____ 6. _____ 7. _____ 8. _____ 9. _____ 10. _____		
_____	1. _____ 2. _____ 3. _____ 4. _____ 5. _____ 6. _____ 7. _____ 8. _____ 9. _____ 10. _____		

LABOR DAY

Year	Favorite Recipes	Recipe Location	Ingredients Needed
	1.		
	2.		
	3.		
	4.		
	5.		
	6.		
	7.		
	8.		
	9.		
	10.		
	1.		
	2.		
	3.		
	4.		
	5.		
	6.		
	7.		
	8.		
	9.		
	10.		
	1.		
	2.		
	3.		
	4.		
	5.		
	6.		
	7.		
	8.		
	9.		
	10.		

THE 95% VEGAN DIET WORKBOOK

LABOR DAY

Year	Favorite Recipes	Recipe Location	Ingredients Needed
_____	1. _____ 2. _____ 3. _____ 4. _____ 5. _____ 6. _____ 7. _____ 8. _____ 9. _____ 10. _____	_____ _____ _____ _____ _____ _____ _____ _____ _____ _____	_____ _____ _____ _____ _____ _____ _____ _____ _____ _____
_____	1. _____ 2. _____ 3. _____ 4. _____ 5. _____ 6. _____ 7. _____ 8. _____ 9. _____ 10. _____	_____ _____ _____ _____ _____ _____ _____ _____ _____ _____	_____ _____ _____ _____ _____ _____ _____ _____ _____ _____

FALL [SEPTEMBER 22 - DECEMBER 20]

SEASONAL FRUITS AND VEGETABLES

apples	artichokes	arugula
Asian pears	avocados	green beans
beets	blackberries	broccoli
Brussels sprouts	burdock	cabbage
carrots	cauliflower	celery
collards	corn	cucumbers
dates	endive	fennel
figs	grapes	guavas
jicama	kale	kiwi
kumquats	leeks	lemons
lettuce	limes	Mandarin oranges
mushrooms	nectarines	okra
onions	oranges	parsnips
peaches	pears	peas
pecans	peppers	persimmons
pistachios	plums	pomegranates
potatoes	quince	raspberries
rhubarb	spinach	strawberries
sweet potatoes	turnips	walnuts

Year	Favorite Recipes	Recipe Location	Ingredients Needed
————	1. _____ 2. _____ 3. _____ 4. _____ 5. _____ 6. _____ 7. _____ 8. _____ 9. _____ 10. _____	_____ _____ _____ _____ _____ _____ _____ _____ _____ _____	_____ _____ _____ _____ _____ _____ _____ _____ _____ _____
————	1. _____ 2. _____ 3. _____ 4. _____ 5. _____ 6. _____ 7. _____ 8. _____ 9. _____ 10. _____	_____ _____ _____ _____ _____ _____ _____ _____ _____ _____	_____ _____ _____ _____ _____ _____ _____ _____ _____ _____
————	1. _____ 2. _____ 3. _____ 4. _____ 5. _____ 6. _____ 7. _____ 8. _____ 9. _____ 10. _____	_____ _____ _____ _____ _____ _____ _____ _____ _____ _____	_____ _____ _____ _____ _____ _____ _____ _____ _____ _____

THE 95% VEGAN DIET WORKBOOK

Year	Favorite Recipes	Recipe Location	Ingredients Needed
_____	1. _____	_____	_____
	2. _____	_____	_____
	3. _____	_____	_____
	4. _____	_____	_____
	5. _____	_____	_____
	6. _____	_____	_____
	7. _____	_____	_____
	8. _____	_____	_____
	9. _____	_____	_____
	10. _____	_____	_____
_____	1. _____	_____	_____
	2. _____	_____	_____
	3. _____	_____	_____
	4. _____	_____	_____
	5. _____	_____	_____
	6. _____	_____	_____
	7. _____	_____	_____
	8. _____	_____	_____
	9. _____	_____	_____
	10. _____	_____	_____

ROSH HASHANAH

Year	Recipes	Recipe Location	Grocery List
	1.		
	2.		
	3.		
	4.		
	5.		
	6.		
	7.		
	8.		
	9.		
	10.		
	1.		
	2.		
	3.		
	4.		
	5.		
	6.		
	7.		
	8.		
	9.		
	10.		
	1.		
	2.		
	3.		
	4.		
	5.		
	6.		
	7.		
	8.		
	9.		
	10.		

ROSH HASHANAH

Year	Recipes	Recipe Location	Grocery List
	1.		
	2.		
	3.		
	4.		
	5.		
	6.		
	7.		
	8.		
	9.		
	10.		
	1.		
	2.		
	3.		
	4.		
	5.		
	6.		
	7.		
	8.		
	9.		
	10.		

OKTOBERFEST

Year	Recipes	Recipe Location	Grocery List
_____	1. _____ 2. _____ 3. _____ 4. _____ 5. _____ 6. _____ 7. _____ 8. _____ 9. _____ 10. _____	_____ _____ _____ _____ _____ _____ _____ _____ _____ _____	_____ _____ _____ _____ _____ _____ _____ _____ _____ _____
_____	1. _____ 2. _____ 3. _____ 4. _____ 5. _____ 6. _____ 7. _____ 8. _____ 9. _____ 10. _____	_____ _____ _____ _____ _____ _____ _____ _____ _____ _____	_____ _____ _____ _____ _____ _____ _____ _____ _____ _____
_____	1. _____ 2. _____ 3. _____ 4. _____ 5. _____ 6. _____ 7. _____ 8. _____ 9. _____ 10. _____	_____ _____ _____ _____ _____ _____ _____ _____ _____ _____	_____ _____ _____ _____ _____ _____ _____ _____ _____ _____

THE 95% VEGAN DIET WORKBOOK

OKTOBERFEST

Year	Recipes	Recipe Location	Grocery List
	1.		
	2.		
	3.		
	4.		
	5.		
	6.		
	7.		
	8.		
	9.		
	10.		
	1.		
	2.		
	3.		
	4.		
	5.		
	6.		
	7.		
	8.		
	9.		
	10.		

HALLOWEEN

Year	Recipes	Recipe Location	Grocery List
_____	1. _____ 2. _____ 3. _____ 4. _____ 5. _____ 6. _____ 7. _____ 8. _____ 9. _____ 10. _____		
_____	1. _____ 2. _____ 3. _____ 4. _____ 5. _____ 6. _____ 7. _____ 8. _____ 9. _____ 10. _____		
_____	1. _____ 2. _____ 3. _____ 4. _____ 5. _____ 6. _____ 7. _____ 8. _____ 9. _____ 10. _____		

HALLOWEEN

Year	Recipes	Recipe Location	Grocery List
	1.		
	2.		
	3.		
	4.		
	5.		
	6.		
	7.		
	8.		
	9.		
	10.		
	1.		
	2.		
	3.		
	4.		
	5.		
	6.		
	7.		
	8.		
	9.		
	10.		

THANKSGIVING

Year	Recipes	Recipe Location	Grocery List
_____	1. _____ 2. _____ 3. _____ 4. _____ 5. _____ 6. _____ 7. _____ 8. _____ 9. _____ 10. _____		
_____	1. _____ 2. _____ 3. _____ 4. _____ 5. _____ 6. _____ 7. _____ 8. _____ 9. _____ 10. _____		
_____	1. _____ 2. _____ 3. _____ 4. _____ 5. _____ 6. _____ 7. _____ 8. _____ 9. _____ 10. _____		

THE 95% VEGAN DIET WORKBOOK

THANKSGIVING

Year	Recipes	Recipe Location	Grocery List
_____	1. _____ 2. _____ 3. _____ 4. _____ 5. _____ 6. _____ 7. _____ 8. _____ 9. _____ 10. _____	_____ _____ _____ _____ _____ _____ _____ _____ _____ _____	_____ _____ _____ _____ _____ _____ _____ _____ _____ _____
_____	1. _____ 2. _____ 3. _____ 4. _____ 5. _____ 6. _____ 7. _____ 8. _____ 9. _____ 10. _____	_____ _____ _____ _____ _____ _____ _____ _____ _____ _____	_____ _____ _____ _____ _____ _____ _____ _____ _____ _____

WINTER [DECEMBER 21 - MARCH 20]

SEASONAL FRUITS AND VEGETABLES

arugula	beets	blood oranges
broccoli	Brussels sprouts	cabbage
carrots	cauliflower	celery
chard	citrons	collards
endive	fava beans	fennel
guavas	jicama	kale
kiwis	leeks	lemons
lettuce	limes	Mandarin oranges
mushrooms	nettles	onions
oranges	parsnips	peanuts
pomelos	potatoes	radishes
rutabagas	spinach	winter squash
sweet potatoes	turnips	

Year	Favorite Recipes	Recipe Location	Ingredients Needed
	1. _____	_____	_____
	2. _____	_____	_____
	3. _____	_____	_____
	4. _____	_____	_____
	5. _____	_____	_____
	6. _____	_____	_____
	7. _____	_____	_____
	8. _____	_____	_____
	9. _____	_____	_____
	10. _____	_____	_____
	1. _____	_____	_____
	2. _____	_____	_____
	3. _____	_____	_____
	4. _____	_____	_____
	5. _____	_____	_____
	6. _____	_____	_____
	7. _____	_____	_____
	8. _____	_____	_____
	9. _____	_____	_____
	10. _____	_____	_____
	1. _____	_____	_____
	2. _____	_____	_____
	3. _____	_____	_____
	4. _____	_____	_____
	5. _____	_____	_____
	6. _____	_____	_____
	7. _____	_____	_____
	8. _____	_____	_____
	9. _____	_____	_____
	10. _____	_____	_____

THE 95% VEGAN DIET WORKBOOK

Year	Favorite Recipes	Recipe Location	Ingredients Needed
_____	1. _____	_____	_____
	2. _____	_____	_____
	3. _____	_____	_____
	4. _____	_____	_____
	5. _____	_____	_____
	6. _____	_____	_____
	7. _____	_____	_____
	8. _____	_____	_____
	9. _____	_____	_____
	10. _____	_____	_____
_____	1. _____	_____	_____
	2. _____	_____	_____
	3. _____	_____	_____
	4. _____	_____	_____
	5. _____	_____	_____
	6. _____	_____	_____
	7. _____	_____	_____
	8. _____	_____	_____
	9. _____	_____	_____
	10. _____	_____	_____

HANUKKAH

Year	Recipes	Recipe Location	Grocery List
	1.		
	2.		
	3.		
	4.		
	5.		
	6.		
	7.		
	8.		
	9.		
	10.		
	1.		
	2.		
	3.		
	4.		
	5.		
	6.		
	7.		
	8.		
	9.		
	10.		
	1.		
	2.		
	3.		
	4.		
	5.		
	6.		
	7.		
	8.		
	9.		
	10.		

THE 95% VEGAN DIET WORKBOOK

HANUKKAH

Year	Recipes	Recipe Location	Grocery List
_____	1. _____ 2. _____ 3. _____ 4. _____ 5. _____ 6. _____ 7. _____ 8. _____ 9. _____ 10. _____		
_____	1. _____ 2. _____ 3. _____ 4. _____ 5. _____ 6. _____ 7. _____ 8. _____ 9. _____ 10. _____		

CHRISTMAS

Year	Recipes	Recipe Location	Grocery List
_____	1. _____ 2. _____ 3. _____ 4. _____ 5. _____ 6. _____ 7. _____ 8. _____ 9. _____ 10. _____		
_____	1. _____ 2. _____ 3. _____ 4. _____ 5. _____ 6. _____ 7. _____ 8. _____ 9. _____ 10. _____		
_____	1. _____ 2. _____ 3. _____ 4. _____ 5. _____ 6. _____ 7. _____ 8. _____ 9. _____ 10. _____		

CHRISTMAS

Year	Recipes	Recipe Location	Grocery List
	1.		
	2.		
	3.		
	4.		
	5.		
	6.		
	7.		
	8.		
	9.		
	10.		
	1.		
	2.		
	3.		
	4.		
	5.		
	6.		
	7.		
	8.		
	9.		
	10.		

KWANZAA

Year	Recipes	Recipe Location	Grocery List
_____	1. _____ 2. _____ 3. _____ 4. _____ 5. _____ 6. _____ 7. _____ 8. _____ 9. _____ 10. _____		
_____	1. _____ 2. _____ 3. _____ 4. _____ 5. _____ 6. _____ 7. _____ 8. _____ 9. _____ 10. _____		
_____	1. _____ 2. _____ 3. _____ 4. _____ 5. _____ 6. _____ 7. _____ 8. _____ 9. _____ 10. _____		

THE 95% VEGAN DIET WORKBOOK

KWANZAA

Year	Recipes	Recipe Location	Grocery List
	1.		
	2.		
	3.		
	4.		
	5.		
	6.		
	7.		
	8.		
	9.		
	10.		
	1.		
	2.		
	3.		
	4.		
	5.		
	6.		
	7.		
	8.		
	9.		
	10.		

NEW YEAR'S DAY

Year	Recipes	Recipe Location	Grocery List
	1.		
	2.		
	3.		
	4.		
	5.		
	6.		
	7.		
	8.		
	9.		
	10.		
	1.		
	2.		
	3.		
	4.		
	5.		
	6.		
	7.		
	8.		
	9.		
	10.		
	1.		
	2.		
	3.		
	4.		
	5.		
	6.		
	7.		
	8.		
	9.		
	10.		

THE 95% VEGAN DIET WORKBOOK

NEW YEAR'S DAY

Year	Recipes	Recipe Location	Grocery List
	1.		
	2.		
	3.		
	4.		
	5.		
	6.		
	7.		
	8.		
	9.		
	10.		
	1.		
	2.		
	3.		
	4.		
	5.		
	6.		
	7.		
	8.		
	9.		
	10.		

CHINESE NEW YEAR

Year	Recipes	Recipe Location	Grocery List
_____	1. _____ 2. _____ 3. _____ 4. _____ 5. _____ 6. _____ 7. _____ 8. _____ 9. _____ 10. _____		
_____	1. _____ 2. _____ 3. _____ 4. _____ 5. _____ 6. _____ 7. _____ 8. _____ 9. _____ 10. _____		
_____	1. _____ 2. _____ 3. _____ 4. _____ 5. _____ 6. _____ 7. _____ 8. _____ 9. _____ 10. _____		

CHINESE NEW YEAR

Year	Recipes	Recipe Location	Grocery List
	1.		
	2.		
	3.		
	4.		
	5.		
	6.		
	7.		
	8.		
	9.		
	10.		
	1.		
	2.		
	3.		
	4.		
	5.		
	6.		
	7.		
	8.		
	9.		
	10.		

SUPER BOWL SUNDAY

Year	Recipes	Recipe Location	Grocery List
	1.		
	2.		
	3.		
	4.		
	5.		
	6.		
	7.		
	8.		
	9.		
	10.		
	1.		
	2.		
	3.		
	4.		
	5.		
	6.		
	7.		
	8.		
	9.		
	10.		
	1.		
	2.		
	3.		
	4.		
	5.		
	6.		
	7.		
	8.		
	9.		
	10.		

THE 95% VEGAN DIET WORKBOOK

SUPER BOWL SUNDAY

Year	Recipes	Recipe Location	Grocery List
	1.		
	2.		
	3.		
	4.		
	5.		
	6.		
	7.		
	8.		
	9.		
	10.		
	1.		
	2.		
	3.		
	4.		
	5.		
	6.		
	7.		
	8.		
	9.		
	10.		

MARDI GRAS

Year	Recipes	Recipe Location	Grocery List
_____	1. _____ 2. _____ 3. _____ 4. _____ 5. _____ 6. _____ 7. _____ 8. _____ 9. _____ 10. _____	_____ _____ _____ _____ _____ _____ _____ _____ _____ _____	_____ _____ _____ _____ _____ _____ _____ _____ _____ _____
_____	1. _____ 2. _____ 3. _____ 4. _____ 5. _____ 6. _____ 7. _____ 8. _____ 9. _____ 10. _____	_____ _____ _____ _____ _____ _____ _____ _____ _____ _____	_____ _____ _____ _____ _____ _____ _____ _____ _____ _____
_____	1. _____ 2. _____ 3. _____ 4. _____ 5. _____ 6. _____ 7. _____ 8. _____ 9. _____ 10. _____	_____ _____ _____ _____ _____ _____ _____ _____ _____ _____	_____ _____ _____ _____ _____ _____ _____ _____ _____ _____

MARDI GRAS

Year	Recipes	Recipe Location	Grocery List
_____	1. _____	_____	_____
	2. _____	_____	_____
	3. _____	_____	_____
	4. _____	_____	_____
	5. _____	_____	_____
	6. _____	_____	_____
	7. _____	_____	_____
	8. _____	_____	_____
	9. _____	_____	_____
	10. _____	_____	_____
_____	1. _____	_____	_____
	2. _____	_____	_____
	3. _____	_____	_____
	4. _____	_____	_____
	5. _____	_____	_____
	6. _____	_____	_____
	7. _____	_____	_____
	8. _____	_____	_____
	9. _____	_____	_____
	10. _____	_____	_____

VALENTINE'S DAY

Year	Recipes	Recipe Location	Grocery List
_____	1. _____ 2. _____ 3. _____ 4. _____ 5. _____ 6. _____ 7. _____ 8. _____ 9. _____ 10. _____	_____ _____ _____ _____ _____ _____ _____ _____ _____ _____	_____ _____ _____ _____ _____ _____ _____ _____ _____ _____
_____	1. _____ 2. _____ 3. _____ 4. _____ 5. _____ 6. _____ 7. _____ 8. _____ 9. _____ 10. _____	_____ _____ _____ _____ _____ _____ _____ _____ _____ _____	_____ _____ _____ _____ _____ _____ _____ _____ _____ _____
_____	1. _____ 2. _____ 3. _____ 4. _____ 5. _____ 6. _____ 7. _____ 8. _____ 9. _____ 10. _____	_____ _____ _____ _____ _____ _____ _____ _____ _____ _____	_____ _____ _____ _____ _____ _____ _____ _____ _____ _____

VALENTINE'S DAY

Year	Recipes	Recipe Location	Grocery List
_____	1. _____ 2. _____ 3. _____ 4. _____ 5. _____ 6. _____ 7. _____ 8. _____ 9. _____ 10. _____		
_____	1. _____ 2. _____ 3. _____ 4. _____ 5. _____ 6. _____ 7. _____ 8. _____ 9. _____ 10. _____		

EXERCISE AND SLEEP

EXERCISE

Here we provide a means for you to track your success in getting your 150 minutes of exercise each week, on average.

Week	Minutes of Exercise	Comments

EXERCISE

Week	Minutes of Exercise	Comments

EXERCISE

Week	Minutes of Exercise	Comments

EXERCISE

Week	Minutes of Exercise	Comments

EXERCISE

Week	Minutes of Exercise	Comments

EXERCISE

Week	Minutes of Exercise	Comments

EXERCISE

Week	Minutes of Exercise	Comments

SLEEP

Here we provide a means for you to track your sleep patterns, should you be having poor sleep. The sleep diary and sleepiness scales are adapted from the National Institutes of Health (NIH), available online at http://science.education.nih.gov/supplements/nih3/sleep/guide/nih_sleep_masters.pdf.

Bring these scales with you to discuss your sleep issues with your physician.

Sleep Diary										
	Friday	Saturday	Sunday	Monday	Tuesday	Wednesday	Thursday	Friday	Saturday	Sunday
Bedtime (to nearest quarter hour)										
Wake time (to nearest quarter hour)										
Total sleep										
Number of awakenings during the night										

	Friday	Saturday	Sunday	Monday	Tuesday	Wednesday	Thursday	Friday	Saturday	Sunday
Bedtime (to nearest quarter hour)										
Wake time (to nearest quarter hour)										
Total sleep										
Number of awakenings during the night										

	Friday	Saturday	Sunday	Monday	Tuesday	Wednesday	Thursday	Friday	Saturday	Sunday
Bedtime (to nearest quarter hour)										
Wake time (to nearest quarter hour)										
Total sleep										
Number of awakenings during the night										

SLEEP

Sleep Diary									
	Friday	Saturday	Sunday	Monday	Tuesday	Wednesday	Thursday	Friday	Saturday	Sunday
Bedtime (to nearest quarter hour)										
Wake time (to nearest quarter hour)										
Total sleep										
Number of awakenings during the night										

	Friday	Saturday	Sunday	Monday	Tuesday	Wednesday	Thursday	Friday	Saturday	Sunday
Bedtime (to nearest quarter hour)										
Wake time (to nearest quarter hour)										
Total sleep										
Number of awakenings during the night										

Sleepiness Scale	
Score	Description
1	Feeling active and vital, alert; wide awake
2	Functioning at high level, but not at peak; able to concentrate
3	Not at full alertness, but responsive and awake
4	Not at peak; let down; slowed down; a little foggy
5	Beginning to lose interest in remaining awake; slowed down; foggy
6	Prefer to be lying down; fighting sleep; woozy
7	Losing struggle to remain awake; sleep onset soon, or asleep

Day/Time	Sleepiness Scale Score	Day/Time	Sleepiness Scale Score	Day/Time	Sleepiness Scale Score
Day:		Day:		Day:	
6:00-7:00 a.m.		6:00-7:00 a.m.		6:00-7:00 a.m.	
10:00 a.m.		10:00 a.m.		10:00 a.m.	
2:00 p.m.		2:00 p.m.		2:00 p.m.	
4:00 p.m.		4:00 p.m.		4:00 p.m.	
7:00 p.m.		7:00 p.m.		7:00 p.m.	
10:00-11:00 p.m.		10:00-11:00 p.m.		10:00-11:00 p.m.	

Day:		Day:		Day:	
6:00-7:00 a.m.		6:00-7:00 a.m.		6:00-7:00 a.m.	
10:00 a.m.		10:00 a.m.		10:00 a.m.	
2:00 p.m.		2:00 p.m.		2:00 p.m.	
4:00 p.m.		4:00 p.m.		4:00 p.m.	
7:00 p.m.		7:00 p.m.		7:00 p.m.	
10:00-11:00 p.m.		10:00-11:00 p.m.		10:00-11:00 p.m.	

Day:		Day:		Day:	
6:00-7:00 a.m.		6:00-7:00 a.m.		6:00-7:00 a.m.	
10:00 a.m.		10:00 a.m.		10:00 a.m.	
2:00 p.m.		2:00 p.m.		2:00 p.m.	
4:00 p.m.		4:00 p.m.		4:00 p.m.	
7:00 p.m.		7:00 p.m.		7:00 p.m.	
10:00-11:00 p.m.		10:00-11:00 p.m.		10:00-11:00 p.m.	

Day:		Day:		Day:	
6:00-7:00 a.m.		6:00-7:00 a.m.		6:00-7:00 a.m.	
10:00 a.m.		10:00 a.m.		10:00 a.m.	
2:00 p.m.		2:00 p.m.		2:00 p.m.	
4:00 p.m.		4:00 p.m.		4:00 p.m.	
7:00 p.m.		7:00 p.m.		7:00 p.m.	
10:00-11:00 p.m.		10:00-11:00 p.m.		10:00-11:00 p.m.	

Day:		Day:		Day:	
6:00-7:00 a.m.		6:00-7:00 a.m.		6:00-7:00 a.m.	
10:00 a.m.		10:00 a.m.		10:00 a.m.	
2:00 p.m.		2:00 p.m.		2:00 p.m.	
4:00 p.m.		4:00 p.m.		4:00 p.m.	
7:00 p.m.		7:00 p.m.		7:00 p.m.	
10:00-11:00 p.m.		10:00-11:00 p.m.		10:00-11:00 p.m.	

THE 95% VEGAN DIET WORKBOOK

Day/Time	Sleepiness Scale Score	Day/Time	Sleepiness Scale Score	Day/Time	Sleepiness Scale Score
Day:		Day:		Day:	
6:00-7:00 a.m.		6:00-7:00 a.m.		6:00-7:00 a.m.	
10:00 a.m.		10:00 a.m.		10:00 a.m.	
2:00 p.m.		2:00 p.m.		2:00 p.m.	
4:00 p.m.		4:00 p.m.		4:00 p.m.	
7:00 p.m.		7:00 p.m.		7:00 p.m.	
10:00-11:00 p.m.		10:00-11:00 p.m.		10:00-11:00 p.m.	

Day/Time	Sleepiness Scale Score	Day/Time	Sleepiness Scale Score	Day/Time	Sleepiness Scale Score
Day:		Day:		Day:	
6:00-7:00 a.m.		6:00-7:00 a.m.		6:00-7:00 a.m.	
10:00 a.m.		10:00 a.m.		10:00 a.m.	
2:00 p.m.		2:00 p.m.		2:00 p.m.	
4:00 p.m.		4:00 p.m.		4:00 p.m.	
7:00 p.m.		7:00 p.m.		7:00 p.m.	
10:00-11:00 p.m.		10:00-11:00 p.m.		10:00-11:00 p.m.	

Day/Time	Sleepiness Scale Score	Day/Time	Sleepiness Scale Score	Day/Time	Sleepiness Scale Score
Day:		Day:		Day:	
6:00-7:00 a.m.		6:00-7:00 a.m.		6:00-7:00 a.m.	
10:00 a.m.		10:00 a.m.		10:00 a.m.	
2:00 p.m.		2:00 p.m.		2:00 p.m.	
4:00 p.m.		4:00 p.m.		4:00 p.m.	
7:00 p.m.		7:00 p.m.		7:00 p.m.	
10:00-11:00 p.m.		10:00-11:00 p.m.		10:00-11:00 p.m.	

Day/Time	Sleepiness Scale Score	Day/Time	Sleepiness Scale Score	Day/Time	Sleepiness Scale Score
Day:		Day:		Day:	
6:00-7:00 a.m.		6:00-7:00 a.m.		6:00-7:00 a.m.	
10:00 a.m.		10:00 a.m.		10:00 a.m.	
2:00 p.m.		2:00 p.m.		2:00 p.m.	
4:00 p.m.		4:00 p.m.		4:00 p.m.	
7:00 p.m.		7:00 p.m.		7:00 p.m.	
10:00-11:00 p.m.		10:00-11:00 p.m.		10:00-11:00 p.m.	

Day/Time	Sleepiness Scale Score	Day/Time	Sleepiness Scale Score	Day/Time	Sleepiness Scale Score
Day:		Day:		Day:	
6:00-7:00 a.m.		6:00-7:00 a.m.		6:00-7:00 a.m.	
10:00 a.m.		10:00 a.m.		10:00 a.m.	
2:00 p.m.		2:00 p.m.		2:00 p.m.	
4:00 p.m.		4:00 p.m.		4:00 p.m.	
7:00 p.m.		7:00 p.m.		7:00 p.m.	
10:00-11:00 p.m.		10:00-11:00 p.m.		10:00-11:00 p.m.	

WEIGHT LOSS

You have plenty of options to decide how best to lose weight as a 95% vegan. You may choose to:

1. Count calories

2. Use the 95% Vegan Diet Food Choices™ Plan

3. Use the 95% Vegan Diet BUC™ Plan, or

4. Develop your own plan

Any of these will work for you, once you identify the appropriate calorie level to lose and maintain your new weight. Also, you can switch from one method to another at any time.

The 95% Vegan Diet Food Choices™ Plan for each calorie level ensures an adequate intake of protein, the amino acid lysine, in particular, since the requirements for other essential amino acids are easily covered within the food choices. Each calorie level also allows for less than 30 percent of calories coming from fat, which is in line with American Heart Association guidelines. If you can cut out even more fat, that is great. If not, at least you know you are within the guidelines established by a highly credible organization.

If you have decided that BMI is an appropriate measurement for you, you can use the table below to determine the maximum amount you can weigh and still have a BMI less than 25.

	5'0"	5'1"	5'2"	5'3"	5'4"	5'5"	5'6"	5'7"	5'8"	5'9"	5'10"	5'11"	6'0"	6'1"	6'2"	6'3"	6'4"
Weight in pounds for BMI<25	127	131	136	140	145	149	153	158	163	167	173	178	183	188	193	198	204

You can also choose to use ideal body weight (IBW) as a goal. To calculate IBW, use the following equation appropriate for your gender:

> Women: 100 lb for the first 5 feet of height, then 5 lb for each additional inch over 5 feet.
> Men: 106 lbs for the first 5 feet of height, then 6 pounds for each additional inch over 5 feet.

If you have a small frame, you may subtract up to 10 percent; if you have a large frame, you may add up to 10 percent.

Choose the number of calories needed to maintain the weight you wish to be (which may or may not be your current weight). This will allow for you to lose the weight while learning new nutritional habits you will need for your lifetime.

Approximate Calories to Maintain Weight								
	Age in Years							
Women	18-25	26-34	35-39	40-45	46-50	51-55	56-62	over 62
100-110lbs	1650	1625	1550	1525	1500	1450	1425	1400
>110-120lbs	1725	1675	1625	1600	1550	1525	1500	1450
>120-130lbs	1800	1750	1700	1675	1625	1600	1550	1525
>130-140lbs	1850	1800	1750	1725	1675	1650	1625	1600
>140-150lbs	1925	1875	1825	1800	1750	1725	1700	1650
>150-160lbs	2000	1950	1900	1850	1825	1800	1750	1725
>160-170lbs	2050	2000	1950	1925	1900	1875	1825	1800
>170-180lbs	2125	2100	2025	2000	1975	1925	1900	1850
Men								
>110-120lbs	1750	1675	1600	1550	1500	1450	1400	1350
>120-130lbs	1975	1900	1825	1800	1725	1675	1625	1575
>130-140lbs	2075	2000	1925	1875	1825	1775	1725	1675
>140-150lbs	2175	2100	2050	2000	1950	1900	1850	1800
>150-160lbs	2300	2225	2150	2100	2050	2000	1950	1900
>160-170lbs	2400	2325	2250	2200	2150	2100	2050	2000
>170-180lbs	2500	2425	2375	2325	2275	2225	2175	2125
>180-190lbs	2625	2550	2475	2425	2375	2325	2275	2225
>190-200lbs	2725	2650	2575	2525	2475	2425	2375	2325
>200-210lbs	2825	2750	2675	2625	2575	2525	2475	2425

You can stop here if you wish to count calories as a 95% vegan, or develop your own system.

If you wish to follow the 95% Vegan Diet Food Choices™ plan, which will provide you all of the proper quantities of protein, carbohydrate, and fat, find your calorie level in the table below and note the number of portions you may eat from each choice list daily. If you wish to use the 95% Vegan Diet BUC™ system, the number of total daily BUCs for each calorie level is at the bottom of the table.

	Calorie Levels														
	1400	1500	1600	1700	1800	1900	2000	2100	2200	2300	2400	2500	2600	2700	2800
Legume	3	4	4	4	4	5	5	6	6	6	7	7	7	7	7
Grain	4	4	5	6	6	6	6	6	6	7	7	7	8	8	8
Vegetable	4	4	4	4	4	4	5	5	5	5	5	5	5	5	6
Fruit	3	3	3	3	3	3	3	3	4	4	4	4	4	5	5
Fat	3	3	3	3	3	3	4	4	4	4	4	4	4	5	5
Dessert	0.5	0.5	0.5	0.5	1	1	1	1	1	1	1	2	2	2	2
Condiment	2	2	2	2	2	2	2	2	3	3	3	3	3	3	3
Choice BUCs per Day	20	22	23	24	26	28	29	30	33	35	37	39	41	43	44

If you find that at the assigned calorie level you are losing more than 2 lb per week after the first few weeks, you are too low on calories. Strive to lose from 0.5 to 1 lb per week based on food intake alone. If you want to lose a bit faster, then increase your activity level. The calories cited for your gender, the weight you want to be, and age, are an *estimate*. While pretty accurate, the table is not perfect in every case. The calories cited for the weight you want to achieve and maintain are making the assumption that you are lightly active on a daily basis. If this is not the case, you may need to increase or decrease the calorie level accordingly. The main thing is that we want to lose fat, not muscle; you can only ensure that if you are losing slowly enough.

If you choose to count calories or use the BUC plan, you will need to be vigilant to ensure you are receiving proper nutrition. Take a look at how the Choice plans break out servings of legumes, grains, fruits, and vegetables for the calorie level you have chosen. These are the number of portions you should still strive to get in each day for good nutrition. Yes, you may have some days of making less than stellar choices; we all do. However, if you strive for optimal nutrition 100 percent of the time and achieve it 95 percent of the time, then you are being *successful*! Remember, you do not have to be *perfect* to be successful.

If you have any health issue for which you are under a doctor's care, you should definitely consult your physician before embarking on any new diet.

Legumes (approximately 110 calories, 8gm protein, 2gm fat, 15gm carbohydrate, 6gm fiber, 1.5BUCs per serving)	Serving Size	Grains (approximately 110 calories, 4gm protein, 1.5gm fat, 20gm carbohydrate, 2gm fiber, 1.5BUCs per serving)	Serving Size	Vegetables (approximately 25calories, 2gm protein, 0gm fat, 4gm carbohydrate, 2gm fiber, 0.25BUCs per serving)	1 cup cooked or 1/2 cup raw except where noted	Fruits (approximately 60 calories, 0 gm protein, 0gm fat, 15gm carbohydrate, 3gm fiber, 1BUC per serving)	Serving Size	Fats (approximately 50 calories, 0gm protein, 6gm fat, 0gm carbohydrate, 0gm fiber per serving)	Serving Size
Soy Milk, regular fat	1 cup	Corn	1 cup	Broccoli		Apples	4 oz, no core	Nuts	1/4 oz
Soy Milk, light	1-1/2 cup	Potato, white	4 oz	Spinach		Oranges	4 oz	Avocado	1 oz
Beans (red, black, white)	1/2 of 15oz can or 3-1/2 oz dried, cooked	Potato, sweet	1-1/2 oz	Carrots		Tangerines	2 oz	Olives	1/2 Tbsp
Chick Peas	1/2 cup cooked	Bread, whole grain	1-1/2 oz	Cabbage		Berries (strawberries, blackberries, blueberries, etc.)	4 oz	Vegan Butter	1/2 Tbsp
Tofu	4 oz	Rice, cooked	1/2 cup	Cauliflower		Dried Fruit	3/4 oz	Oils	1/2 Tbsp
Split Peas	1/2 cup cooked	Pasta, cooked	3 oz	Tomatoes		Watermelon	8 oz	Flax Seed	1/2 Tbsp
Soy Tempeh	2 oz	Noodles, cooked	3 oz	Summer Squash (yellow, zucchini)		Peaches/Nectarines	6 oz		
Soy Yogurt	4 oz	Grain Flours (wheat, rye, oat, etc.)	1/4 cup	Cucumber, 1 medium		Cherries	3 oz		

Legumes (approximately 110 calories, 8gm protein, 2gm fat, 15gm carbohydrate, 6gm fiber, 1.5BUCs per serving)	Serving Size	Grains (approximately 110 calories, 4gm protein, 1.5gm fat, 20gm carbohydrate, 2gm fiber, 1.5BUCs per serving)	Serving Size	Vegetables (approximately 25calories, 2gm protein, 0gm fat, 4gm carbohydrate, 2gm fiber, 0.25BUCs per serving)	1 cup cooked or 1/2 cup raw except where noted	Fruits (approximately 60 calories, 0 gm protein, 0gm fat, 15gm carbohydrate, 3gm fiber, 1BUC per serving)	Serving Size	Fats (approximately 50 calories, 0gm protein, 6gm fat, 0gm carbohydrate, 0gm fiber per serving)	Serving Size
Soy Beans (Edamame in Shell)	4 oz	Winter Squash (acorn, butternut, etc.)	10 oz cooked			Grapes	3 oz		
Soy Beans, shelled	3 oz	Pretzels	1 oz			Banana	2-1/2 oz		
Green Peas	5 oz	Popcorn, popped	4 cups						
TVP (texturized vegetable protein)	1/3 cup dry								
Nutritional Yeast Flakes	1/2 cup cooked								
Legume Flours (soy, garbanzo, etc.)	1/4 cup								

Desserts (approximately 200 calories, 2gm protein, 10gm fat, 26gm carbohydrate, 1gm fiber, 3 BUCs per serving)		Condiments (approximately 50 calories, macronutrient content varies, 1BUC per serving)	Serving Size	Misc.	Choices per Serving	BUCs per serving			
Do not exceed calorie amount		Catsup	4 Tbsp	Potato Chips, 1oz.	1 grain, 1 fat	3			
		Sugar	1 Tbsp	Granola Bar, 1	1 grain, 1 fat	3			
Free Foods		Honey	2-1/2 tsp	Biscuit, 1 medium (2-1/2 inches wide)	1 grain, 1/2 fat	2			
Vegetable bouillon		Sugar-free maple syrup	4 Tbsp						
Dill pickles		Non-dairy coffee creamer	2 Tbsp						
Spices									
Herbs									
Coffee or tea, black									
Diet sodas									
Lemon juice									
Lime juice									

Practice before starting by making a seven-day meal plan.

THE 95% VEGAN DIET WORKBOOK

7 Day Meal Plan for 95% Vegan Diet Calorie Counting™

Calories per day: _____

Day:	Breakfast	Calories	Lunch	Calories	Dinner	Calories	Snack	Calories	Snack	Calories	Snack	Calories
1												
2												
3												
4												
5												
6												
7												

7 Day Meal Plan for the 95% Vegan Diet Food Choice Plan™

Choices per Day

Legume: _____ Grain: _____ Fruit: _____ Vegetable: _____ Fat: _____ Dessert: _____ Condiment: _____

Day:	Breakfast	Choices	Lunch	Choices	Dinner	Choices	Snack	Choices	Snack	Choices	Snack	Choices
1												
2												
3												
4												
5												
6												
7												

7 Day Meal Plan for the 95% Vegan Diet BUC Plan™

BUCs per day: _____

Day:	Breakfast	BUCs	Lunch	BUCs	Dinner	BUCs	Snack	BUCs	Snack	BUCs	Snack	BUCs	Total BUCS
1													
2													
3													
4													
5													
6													
7													

PREDIABETES AND TYPE 2 DIABETES MELLITUS

The goal here is to discover any *patterns* in your blood glucose measurements for which adjustments may be needed. This is *not* a pass/fail test; it is simply *checking* to see where you are in terms of control.

Date:		Day of Week:				
Fasting (before breakfast)	2 hrs after breakfast	Before lunch	2 hrs after lunch	Before supper	2 hrs after supper	Bedtime

Date:		Day of Week:				
Fasting (before breakfast)	2 hrs after breakfast	Before lunch	2 hrs after lunch	Before supper	2 hrs after supper	Bedtime

Date:		Day of Week:				
Fasting (before breakfast)	2 hrs after breakfast	Before lunch	2 hrs after lunch	Before supper	2 hrs after supper	Bedtime

Date:		Day of Week:				
Fasting (before breakfast)	2 hrs after breakfast	Before lunch	2 hrs after lunch	Before supper	2 hrs after supper	Bedtime

Date:		Day of Week:				
Fasting (before breakfast)	2 hrs after breakfast	Before lunch	2 hrs after lunch	Before supper	2 hrs after supper	Bedtime

Date:		Day of Week:				
Fasting (before breakfast)	2 hrs after breakfast	Before lunch	2 hrs after lunch	Before supper	2 hrs after supper	Bedtime

Date:		Day of Week:				
Fasting (before breakfast)	2 hrs after breakfast	Before lunch	2 hrs after lunch	Before supper	2 hrs after supper	Bedtime

Date:		Day of Week:				
Fasting (before breakfast)	2 hrs after breakfast	Before lunch	2 hrs after lunch	Before supper	2 hrs after supper	Bedtime

Date:		Day of Week:				
Fasting (before breakfast)	2 hrs after breakfast	Before lunch	2 hrs after lunch	Before supper	2 hrs after supper	Bedtime

Date:		Day of Week:				
Fasting (before breakfast)	2 hrs after breakfast	Before lunch	2 hrs after lunch	Before supper	2 hrs after supper	Bedtime

Date:		Day of Week:				
Fasting (before breakfast)	2 hrs after breakfast	Before lunch	2 hrs after lunch	Before supper	2 hrs after supper	Bedtime

THE 95% VEGAN DIET WORKBOOK

Date:		Day of Week:				
Fasting (before breakfast)	2 hrs after breakfast	Before lunch	2 hrs after lunch	Before supper	2 hrs after supper	Bedtime

Date:		Day of Week:				
Fasting (before breakfast)	2 hrs after breakfast	Before lunch	2 hrs after lunch	Before supper	2 hrs after supper	Bedtime

Date:		Day of Week:				
Fasting (before breakfast)	2 hrs after breakfast	Before lunch	2 hrs after lunch	Before supper	2 hrs after supper	Bedtime

Date:		Day of Week:				
Fasting (before breakfast)	2 hrs after breakfast	Before lunch	2 hrs after lunch	Before supper	2 hrs after supper	Bedtime

Date:		Day of Week:				
Fasting (before breakfast)	2 hrs after breakfast	Before lunch	2 hrs after lunch	Before supper	2 hrs after supper	Bedtime

Date:		Day of Week:				
Fasting (before breakfast)	2 hrs after breakfast	Before lunch	2 hrs after lunch	Before supper	2 hrs after supper	Bedtime

Date:		Day of Week:				
Fasting (before breakfast)	2 hrs after breakfast	Before lunch	2 hrs after lunch	Before supper	2 hrs after supper	Bedtime

Date:		Day of Week:				
Fasting (before breakfast)	2 hrs after breakfast	Before lunch	2 hrs after lunch	Before supper	2 hrs after supper	Bedtime

Date:		Day of Week:				
Fasting (before breakfast)	2 hrs after breakfast	Before lunch	2 hrs after lunch	Before supper	2 hrs after supper	Bedtime

Date:		Day of Week:				
Fasting (before breakfast)	2 hrs after breakfast	Before lunch	2 hrs after lunch	Before supper	2 hrs after supper	Bedtime

Date:		Day of Week:				
Fasting (before breakfast)	2 hrs after breakfast	Before lunch	2 hrs after lunch	Before supper	2 hrs after supper	Bedtime

Date:		Day of Week:				
Fasting (before breakfast)	2 hrs after breakfast	Before lunch	2 hrs after lunch	Before supper	2 hrs after supper	Bedtime

Date:		Day of Week:				
Fasting (before breakfast)	2 hrs after breakfast	Before lunch	2 hrs after lunch	Before supper	2 hrs after supper	Bedtime

Date:		Day of Week:				
Fasting (before breakfast)	2 hrs after breakfast	Before lunch	2 hrs after lunch	Before supper	2 hrs after supper	Bedtime

Date:		Day of Week:				
Fasting (before breakfast)	2 hrs after breakfast	Before lunch	2 hrs after lunch	Before supper	2 hrs after supper	Bedtime

Date:		Day of Week:				
Fasting (before breakfast)	2 hrs after breakfast	Before lunch	2 hrs after lunch	Before supper	2 hrs after supper	Bedtime

Date:		Day of Week:				
Fasting (before breakfast)	2 hrs after breakfast	Before lunch	2 hrs after lunch	Before supper	2 hrs after supper	Bedtime

BECOME YOUR OWN SCIENTIST

WHAT IS GOOD SCIENCE?

In the book, we discussed at length what makes good science. Here we provide a means for you to objectively assess whether or not a medicine or supplement has good science to support a positive risk/benefit profile. You can also use these pages to assess whether there is good science behind individual foods. For example, we now have an abundance of claims that certain foods have medicinal benefits. Use these pages to assess what type of science, if any, there is to support the claims.

Good Science Checklist	
Product name:	
Number of studies completed in humans:	
Studies published in:	████████████████████████████
Journal:	
Journal:	
Journal:	
Journal:	
Journal:	

Complete the following checklist for each study published.

Study Title:	
Study sponsor(s):	
Human population:	████████████████████████████
Average age of study subjects:	
Age range:	
Both genders equally? (Y/N)	
Race/ethnicities studied	
Number of study subjects (people)	
Statistical powering %:	
Length of study:	
Study design: parallel? crossover?	
Double-blind?	
Prospective? (Y/N)	
Randomized? (Y/N)	
What controls were in place?	
Hypothesis stated? (Y/N)	
Comparator(s)	
Outcomes	
Statistically significant?	
Clinically significant?	
Side effects observed	
Safety issues, if any	
Did the study population represent YOU (age, gender, ethnicity, etc.)?	
In your judgment, does this study support you taking this product? Why or why not?	

THE 95% VEGAN DIET WORKBOOK   133

Complete the following checklist for each study published.

Study Title:	
Study sponsor(s):	
Human population:	
Average age of study subjects:	
Age range:	
Both genders equally? (Y/N)	
Race/ethnicities studied	
Number of study subjects (people)	
Statistical powering %:	
Length of study:	
Study design: parallel? crossover?	
Double-blind?	
Prospective? (Y/N)	
Randomized? (Y/N)	
What controls were in place?	
Hypothesis stated? (Y/N)	
Comparator(s)	
Outcomes	
Statistically significant?	
Clinically significant?	
Side effects observed	
Safety issues, if any	
Did the study population represent YOU (age, gender, ethnicity, etc.)?	
In your judgment, does this study support you taking this product? Why or why not?	

Complete the following checklist for each study published.

Study Title:	
Study sponsor(s):	
Human population:	
Average age of study subjects:	
Age range:	
Both genders equally? (Y/N)	
Race/ethnicities studied	
Number of study subjects (people)	
Statistical powering %:	
Length of study:	
Study design: parallel? crossover?	
Double-blind?	
Prospective? (Y/N)	
Randomized? (Y/N)	
What controls were in place?	
Hypothesis stated? (Y/N)	
Comparator(s)	
Outcomes	
Statistically significant?	
Clinically significant?	
Side effects observed	
Safety issues, if any	
Did the study population represent YOU (age, gender, ethnicity, etc.)?	
In your judgment, does this study support you taking this product? Why or why not?	

THE 95% VEGAN DIET WORKBOOK

Complete the following checklist for each study published.

Study Title:	
Study sponsor(s):	
Human population:	
Average age of study subjects:	
Age range:	
Both genders equally? (Y/N)	
Race/ethnicities studied	
Number of study subjects (people)	
Statistical powering %:	
Length of study:	
Study design: parallel? crossover?	
Double-blind?	
Prospective? (Y/N)	
Randomized? (Y/N)	
What controls were in place?	
Hypothesis stated? (Y/N)	
Comparator(s)	
Outcomes	
Statistically significant?	
Clinically significant?	
Side effects observed	
Safety issues, if any	
Did the study population represent YOU (age, gender, ethnicity, etc.)?	
In your judgment, does this study support you taking this product? Why or why not?	

Complete the following checklist for each study published.

Study Title:	
Study sponsor(s):	
Human population:	
Average age of study subjects:	
Age range:	
Both genders equally? (Y/N)	
Race/ethnicities studied	
Number of study subjects (people)	
Statistical powering %:	
Length of study:	
Study design: parallel? crossover?	
Double-blind?	
Prospective? (Y/N)	
Randomized? (Y/N)	
What controls were in place?	
Hypothesis stated? (Y/N)	
Comparator(s)	
Outcomes	
Statistically significant?	
Clinically significant?	
Side effects observed	
Safety issues, if any	
Did the study population represent YOU (age, gender, ethnicity, etc.)?	
In your judgment, does this study support you taking this product? Why or why not?	

Good Science Checklist	
Product name:	
Number of studies completed in humans:	
Studies published in:	
Journal:	
Journal:	
Journal:	
Journal:	
Journal:	

Complete the following checklist for each study published.

Study Title:	
Study sponsor(s):	
Human population:	
Average age of study subjects:	
Age range:	
Both genders equally? (Y/N)	
Race/ethnicities studied	
Number of study subjects (people)	
Statistical powering %:	
Length of study:	
Study design: parallel? crossover?	
Double-blind?	
Prospective? (Y/N)	
Randomized? (Y/N)	
What controls were in place?	
Hypothesis stated? (Y/N)	
Comparator(s)	
Outcomes	
Statistically significant?	
Clinically significant?	
Side effects observed	
Safety issues, if any	
Did the study population represent YOU (age, gender, ethnicity, etc.)?	
In your judgment, does this study support you taking this product? Why or why not?	

Complete the following checklist for each study published.

Study Title:	
Study sponsor(s):	
Human population:	
Average age of study subjects:	
Age range:	
Both genders equally? (Y/N)	
Race/ethnicities studied	
Number of study subjects (people)	
Statistical powering %:	
Length of study:	
Study design: parallel? crossover?	
Double-blind?	
Prospective? (Y/N)	
Randomized? (Y/N)	
What controls were in place?	
Hypothesis stated? (Y/N)	
Comparator(s)	
Outcomes	
Statistically significant?	
Clinically significant?	
Side effects observed	
Safety issues, if any	
Did the study population represent YOU (age, gender, ethnicity, etc.)?	
In your judgment, does this study support you taking this product? Why or why not?	

THE 95% VEGAN DIET WORKBOOK

Complete the following checklist for each study published.

Study Title:	
Study sponsor(s):	
Human population:	
Average age of study subjects:	
Age range:	
Both genders equally? (Y/N)	
Race/ethnicities studied	
Number of study subjects (people)	
Statistical powering %:	
Length of study:	
Study design: parallel? crossover?	
Double-blind?	
Prospective? (Y/N)	
Randomized? (Y/N)	
What controls were in place?	
Hypothesis stated? (Y/N)	
Comparator(s)	
Outcomes	
Statistically significant?	
Clinically significant?	
Side effects observed	
Safety issues, if any	
Did the study population represent YOU (age, gender, ethnicity, etc.)?	
In your judgment, does this study support you taking this product? Why or why not?	

Complete the following checklist for each study published.

Study Title:	
Study sponsor(s):	
Human population:	
Average age of study subjects:	
Age range:	
Both genders equally? (Y/N)	
Race/ethnicities studied	
Number of study subjects (people)	
Statistical powering %:	
Length of study:	
Study design: parallel? crossover?	
Double-blind?	
Prospective? (Y/N)	
Randomized? (Y/N)	
What controls were in place?	
Hypothesis stated? (Y/N)	
Comparator(s)	
Outcomes	
Statistically significant?	
Clinically significant?	
Side effects observed	
Safety issues, if any	
Did the study population represent YOU (age, gender, ethnicity, etc.)?	
In your judgment, does this study support you taking this product? Why or why not?	

THE 95% VEGAN DIET WORKBOOK

Complete the following checklist for each study published.

Study Title:	
Study sponsor(s):	
Human population:	
Average age of study subjects:	
Age range:	
Both genders equally? (Y/N)	
Race/ethnicities studied	
Number of study subjects (people)	
Statistical powering %:	
Length of study:	
Study design: parallel? crossover?	
Double-blind?	
Prospective? (Y/N)	
Randomized? (Y/N)	
What controls were in place?	
Hypothesis stated? (Y/N)	
Comparator(s)	
Outcomes	
Statistically significant?	
Clinically significant?	
Side effects observed	
Safety issues, if any	
Did the study population represent YOU (age, gender, ethnicity, etc.)?	
In your judgment, does this study support you taking this product? Why or why not?	

Good Science Checklist	
Product name:	
Number of studies completed in humans:	
Studies published in:	
Journal:	
Journal:	
Journal:	
Journal:	
Journal:	

Complete the following checklist for each study published.

Study Title:	
Study sponsor(s):	
Human population:	
Average age of study subjects:	
Age range:	
Both genders equally? (Y/N)	
Race/ethnicities studied	
Number of study subjects (people)	
Statistical powering %:	
Length of study:	
Study design: parallel? crossover?	
Double-blind?	
Prospective? (Y/N)	
Randomized? (Y/N)	
What controls were in place?	
Hypothesis stated? (Y/N)	
Comparator(s)	
Outcomes	
Statistically significant?	
Clinically significant?	
Side effects observed	
Safety issues, if any	
Did the study population represent YOU (age, gender, ethnicity, etc.)?	
In your judgment, does this study support you taking this product? Why or why not?	

THE 95% VEGAN DIET WORKBOOK

Complete the following checklist for each study published.

Study Title:	
Study sponsor(s):	
Human population:	
Average age of study subjects:	
Age range:	
Both genders equally? (Y/N)	
Race/ethnicities studied	
Number of study subjects (people)	
Statistical powering %:	
Length of study:	
Study design: parallel? crossover?	
Double-blind?	
Prospective? (Y/N)	
Randomized? (Y/N)	
What controls were in place?	
Hypothesis stated? (Y/N)	
Comparator(s)	
Outcomes	
Statistically significant?	
Clinically significant?	
Side effects observed	
Safety issues, if any	
Did the study population represent YOU (age, gender, ethnicity, etc.)?	
In your judgment, does this study support you taking this product? Why or why not?	

Complete the following checklist for each study published.

Study Title:	
Study sponsor(s):	
Human population:	
Average age of study subjects:	
Age range:	
Both genders equally? (Y/N)	
Race/ethnicities studied	
Number of study subjects (people)	
Statistical powering %:	
Length of study:	
Study design: parallel? crossover?	
Double-blind?	
Prospective? (Y/N)	
Randomized? (Y/N)	
What controls were in place?	
Hypothesis stated? (Y/N)	
Comparator(s)	
Outcomes	
Statistically significant?	
Clinically significant?	
Side effects observed	
Safety issues, if any	
Did the study population represent YOU (age, gender, ethnicity, etc.)?	
In your judgment, does this study support you taking this product? Why or why not?	

Complete the following checklist for each study published.

Study Title:	
Study sponsor(s):	
Human population:	
Average age of study subjects:	
Age range:	
Both genders equally? (Y/N)	
Race/ethnicities studied	
Number of study subjects (people)	
Statistical powering %:	
Length of study:	
Study design: parallel? crossover?	
Double-blind?	
Prospective? (Y/N)	
Randomized? (Y/N)	
What controls were in place?	
Hypothesis stated? (Y/N)	
Comparator(s)	
Outcomes	
Statistically significant?	
Clinically significant?	
Side effects observed	
Safety issues, if any	
Did the study population represent YOU (age, gender, ethnicity, etc.)?	
In your judgment, does this study support you taking this product? Why or why not?	

Complete the following checklist for each study published.

Study Title:	
Study sponsor(s):	
Human population:	
Average age of study subjects:	
Age range:	
Both genders equally? (Y/N)	
Race/ethnicities studied	
Number of study subjects (people)	
Statistical powering %:	
Length of study:	
Study design: parallel? crossover?	
Double-blind?	
Prospective? (Y/N)	
Randomized? (Y/N)	
What controls were in place?	
Hypothesis stated? (Y/N)	
Comparator(s)	
Outcomes	
Statistically significant?	
Clinically significant?	
Side effects observed	
Safety issues, if any	
Did the study population represent YOU (age, gender, ethnicity, etc.)?	
In your judgment, does this study support you taking this product? Why or why not?	

THE 95% VEGAN DIET WORKBOOK

Good Science Checklist	
Product name:	
Number of studies completed in humans:	
Studies published in:	
Journal:	
Journal:	
Journal:	
Journal:	
Journal:	

Complete the following checklist for each study published.

Study Title:	
Study sponsor(s):	
Human population:	
Average age of study subjects:	
Age range:	
Both genders equally? (Y/N)	
Race/ethnicities studied	
Number of study subjects (people)	
Statistical powering %:	
Length of study:	
Study design: parallel? crossover?	
Double-blind?	
Prospective? (Y/N)	
Randomized? (Y/N)	
What controls were in place?	
Hypothesis stated? (Y/N)	
Comparator(s)	
Outcomes	
Statistically significant?	
Clinically significant?	
Side effects observed	
Safety issues, if any	
Did the study population represent YOU (age, gender, ethnicity, etc.)?	
In your judgment, does this study support you taking this product? Why or why not?	

Complete the following checklist for each study published.

Study Title:	
Study sponsor(s):	
Human population:	
Average age of study subjects:	
Age range:	
Both genders equally? (Y/N)	
Race/ethnicities studied	
Number of study subjects (people)	
Statistical powering %:	
Length of study:	
Study design: parallel? crossover?	
Double-blind?	
Prospective? (Y/N)	
Randomized? (Y/N)	
What controls were in place?	
Hypothesis stated? (Y/N)	
Comparator(s)	
Outcomes	
Statistically significant?	
Clinically significant?	
Side effects observed	
Safety issues, if any	
Did the study population represent YOU (age, gender, ethnicity, etc.)?	
In your judgment, does this study support you taking this product? Why or why not?	

THE 95% VEGAN DIET WORKBOOK

Complete the following checklist for each study published.

Study Title:	
Study sponsor(s):	
Human population:	
Average age of study subjects:	
Age range:	
Both genders equally? (Y/N)	
Race/ethnicities studied	
Number of study subjects (people)	
Statistical powering %:	
Length of study:	
Study design: parallel? crossover?	
Double-blind?	
Prospective? (Y/N)	
Randomized? (Y/N)	
What controls were in place?	
Hypothesis stated? (Y/N)	
Comparator(s)	
Outcomes	
Statistically significant?	
Clinically significant?	
Side effects observed	
Safety issues, if any	
Did the study population represent YOU (age, gender, ethnicity, etc.)?	
In your judgment, does this study support you taking this product? Why or why not?	

Complete the following checklist for each study published.

Study Title:	
Study sponsor(s):	
Human population:	
Average age of study subjects:	
Age range:	
Both genders equally? (Y/N)	
Race/ethnicities studied	
Number of study subjects (people)	
Statistical powering %:	
Length of study:	
Study design: parallel? crossover?	
Double-blind?	
Prospective? (Y/N)	
Randomized? (Y/N)	
What controls were in place?	
Hypothesis stated? (Y/N)	
Comparator(s)	
Outcomes	
Statistically significant?	
Clinically significant?	
Side effects observed	
Safety issues, if any	
Did the study population represent YOU (age, gender, ethnicity, etc.)?	
In your judgment, does this study support you taking this product? Why or why not?	

THE 95% VEGAN DIET WORKBOOK

Complete the following checklist for each study published.

Study Title:	
Study sponsor(s):	
Human population:	
Average age of study subjects:	
Age range:	
Both genders equally? (Y/N)	
Race/ethnicities studied	
Number of study subjects (people)	
Statistical powering %:	
Length of study:	
Study design: parallel? crossover?	
Double-blind?	
Prospective? (Y/N)	
Randomized? (Y/N)	
What controls were in place?	
Hypothesis stated? (Y/N)	
Comparator(s)	
Outcomes	
Statistically significant?	
Clinically significant?	
Side effects observed	
Safety issues, if any	
Did the study population represent YOU (age, gender, ethnicity, etc.)?	
In your judgment, does this study support you taking this product? Why or why not?	

Good Science Checklist	
Product name:	
Number of studies completed in humans:	
Studies published in:	██████████████████████
Journal:	
Journal:	
Journal:	
Journal:	
Journal:	

Complete the following checklist for each study published.

Study Title:	
Study sponsor(s):	
Human population:	██████████████████████
Average age of study subjects:	
Age range:	
Both genders equally? (Y/N)	
Race/ethnicities studied	
Number of study subjects (people)	
Statistical powering %:	
Length of study:	
Study design: parallel? crossover?	
Double-blind?	
Prospective? (Y/N)	
Randomized? (Y/N)	
What controls were in place?	
Hypothesis stated? (Y/N)	
Comparator(s)	
Outcomes	
Statistically significant?	
Clinically significant?	
Side effects observed	
Safety issues, if any	
Did the study population represent YOU (age, gender, ethnicity, etc.)?	
In your judgment, does this study support you taking this product? Why or why not?	

Complete the following checklist for each study published.

Study Title:	
Study sponsor(s):	
Human population:	
Average age of study subjects:	
Age range:	
Both genders equally? (Y/N)	
Race/ethnicities studied	
Number of study subjects (people)	
Statistical powering %:	
Length of study:	
Study design: parallel? crossover?	
Double-blind?	
Prospective? (Y/N)	
Randomized? (Y/N)	
What controls were in place?	
Hypothesis stated? (Y/N)	
Comparator(s)	
Outcomes	
Statistically significant?	
Clinically significant?	
Side effects observed	
Safety issues, if any	
Did the study population represent YOU (age, gender, ethnicity, etc.)?	
In your judgment, does this study support you taking this product? Why or why not?	

Complete the following checklist for each study published.

Study Title:	
Study sponsor(s):	
Human population:	
Average age of study subjects:	
Age range:	
Both genders equally? (Y/N)	
Race/ethnicities studied	
Number of study subjects (people)	
Statistical powering %:	
Length of study:	
Study design: parallel? crossover?	
Double-blind?	
Prospective? (Y/N)	
Randomized? (Y/N)	
What controls were in place?	
Hypothesis stated? (Y/N)	
Comparator(s)	
Outcomes	
Statistically significant?	
Clinically significant?	
Side effects observed	
Safety issues, if any	
Did the study population represent YOU (age, gender, ethnicity, etc.)?	
In your judgment, does this study support you taking this product? Why or why not?	

THE 95% VEGAN DIET WORKBOOK   155

Complete the following checklist for each study published.

Study Title:	
Study sponsor(s):	
Human population:	
Average age of study subjects:	
Age range:	
Both genders equally? (Y/N)	
Race/ethnicities studied	
Number of study subjects (people)	
Statistical powering %:	
Length of study:	
Study design: parallel? crossover?	
Double-blind?	
Prospective? (Y/N)	
Randomized? (Y/N)	
What controls were in place?	
Hypothesis stated? (Y/N)	
Comparator(s)	
Outcomes	
Statistically significant?	
Clinically significant?	
Side effects observed	
Safety issues, if any	
Did the study population represent YOU (age, gender, ethnicity, etc.)?	
In your judgment, does this study support you taking this product? Why or why not?	

Complete the following checklist for each study published.

Study Title:	
Study sponsor(s):	
Human population:	
Average age of study subjects:	
Age range:	
Both genders equally? (Y/N)	
Race/ethnicities studied	
Number of study subjects (people)	
Statistical powering %:	
Length of study:	
Study design: parallel? crossover?	
Double-blind?	
Prospective? (Y/N)	
Randomized? (Y/N)	
What controls were in place?	
Hypothesis stated? (Y/N)	
Comparator(s)	
Outcomes	
Statistically significant?	
Clinically significant?	
Side effects observed	
Safety issues, if any	
Did the study population represent YOU (age, gender, ethnicity, etc.)?	
In your judgment, does this study support you taking this product? Why or why not?	

THE 95% VEGAN DIET WORKBOOK

Good Science Checklist	
Product name:	
Number of studies completed in humans:	
Studies published in:	
Journal:	
Journal:	
Journal:	
Journal:	
Journal:	

Complete the following checklist for each study published.

Study Title:	
Study sponsor(s):	
Human population:	
Average age of study subjects:	
Age range:	
Both genders equally? (Y/N)	
Race/ethnicities studied	
Number of study subjects (people)	
Statistical powering %:	
Length of study:	
Study design: parallel? crossover?	
Double-blind?	
Prospective? (Y/N)	
Randomized? (Y/N)	
What controls were in place?	
Hypothesis stated? (Y/N)	
Comparator(s)	
Outcomes	
Statistically significant?	
Clinically significant?	
Side effects observed	
Safety issues, if any	
Did the study population represent YOU (age, gender, ethnicity, etc.)?	
In your judgment, does this study support you taking this product? Why or why not?	

Complete the following checklist for each study published.

Study Title:	
Study sponsor(s):	
Human population:	
Average age of study subjects:	
Age range:	
Both genders equally? (Y/N)	
Race/ethnicities studied	
Number of study subjects (people)	
Statistical powering %:	
Length of study:	
Study design: parallel? crossover?	
Double-blind?	
Prospective? (Y/N)	
Randomized? (Y/N)	
What controls were in place?	
Hypothesis stated? (Y/N)	
Comparator(s)	
Outcomes	
Statistically significant?	
Clinically significant?	
Side effects observed	
Safety issues, if any	
Did the study population represent YOU (age, gender, ethnicity, etc.)?	
In your judgment, does this study support you taking this product? Why or why not?	

THE 95% VEGAN DIET WORKBOOK

Complete the following checklist for each study published.

Study Title:	
Study sponsor(s):	
Human population:	
Average age of study subjects:	
Age range:	
Both genders equally? (Y/N)	
Race/ethnicities studied	
Number of study subjects (people)	
Statistical powering %:	
Length of study:	
Study design: parallel? crossover?	
Double-blind?	
Prospective? (Y/N)	
Randomized? (Y/N)	
What controls were in place?	
Hypothesis stated? (Y/N)	
Comparator(s)	
Outcomes	
Statistically significant?	
Clinically significant?	
Side effects observed	
Safety issues, if any	
Did the study population represent YOU (age, gender, ethnicity, etc.)?	
In your judgment, does this study support you taking this product? Why or why not?	

Complete the following checklist for each study published.

Study Title:	
Study sponsor(s):	
Human population:	
Average age of study subjects:	
Age range:	
Both genders equally? (Y/N)	
Race/ethnicities studied	
Number of study subjects (people)	
Statistical powering %:	
Length of study:	
Study design: parallel? crossover?	
Double-blind?	
Prospective? (Y/N)	
Randomized? (Y/N)	
What controls were in place?	
Hypothesis stated? (Y/N)	
Comparator(s)	
Outcomes	
Statistically significant?	
Clinically significant?	
Side effects observed	
Safety issues, if any	
Did the study population represent YOU (age, gender, ethnicity, etc.)?	
In your judgment, does this study support you taking this product? Why or why not?	

Complete the following checklist for each study published.

Study Title:	
Study sponsor(s):	
Human population:	
Average age of study subjects:	
Age range:	
Both genders equally? (Y/N)	
Race/ethnicities studied	
Number of study subjects (people)	
Statistical powering %:	
Length of study:	
Study design: parallel? crossover?	
Double-blind?	
Prospective? (Y/N)	
Randomized? (Y/N)	
What controls were in place?	
Hypothesis stated? (Y/N)	
Comparator(s)	
Outcomes	
Statistically significant?	
Clinically significant?	
Side effects observed	
Safety issues, if any	
Did the study population represent YOU (age, gender, ethnicity, etc.)?	
In your judgment, does this study support you taking this product? Why or why not?	

Good Science Checklist	
Product name:	
Number of studies completed in humans:	
Studies published in:	
Journal:	
Journal:	
Journal:	
Journal:	
Journal:	

Complete the following checklist for each study published.

Study Title:	
Study sponsor(s):	
Human population:	
Average age of study subjects:	
Age range:	
Both genders equally? (Y/N)	
Race/ethnicities studied	
Number of study subjects (people)	
Statistical powering %:	
Length of study:	
Study design: parallel? crossover?	
Double-blind?	
Prospective? (Y/N)	
Randomized? (Y/N)	
What controls were in place?	
Hypothesis stated? (Y/N)	
Comparator(s)	
Outcomes	
Statistically significant?	
Clinically significant?	
Side effects observed	
Safety issues, if any	
Did the study population represent YOU (age, gender, ethnicity, etc.)?	
In your judgment, does this study support you taking this product? Why or why not?	

Complete the following checklist for each study published.

Study Title:	
Study sponsor(s):	
Human population:	
Average age of study subjects:	
Age range:	
Both genders equally? (Y/N)	
Race/ethnicities studied	
Number of study subjects (people)	
Statistical powering %:	
Length of study:	
Study design: parallel? crossover?	
Double-blind?	
Prospective? (Y/N)	
Randomized? (Y/N)	
What controls were in place?	
Hypothesis stated? (Y/N)	
Comparator(s)	
Outcomes	
Statistically significant?	
Clinically significant?	
Side effects observed	
Safety issues, if any	
Did the study population represent YOU (age, gender, ethnicity, etc.)?	
In your judgment, does this study support you taking this product? Why or why not?	

Complete the following checklist for each study published.

Study Title:	
Study sponsor(s):	
Human population:	
Average age of study subjects:	
Age range:	
Both genders equally? (Y/N)	
Race/ethnicities studied	
Number of study subjects (people)	
Statistical powering %:	
Length of study:	
Study design: parallel? crossover?	
Double-blind?	
Prospective? (Y/N)	
Randomized? (Y/N)	
What controls were in place?	
Hypothesis stated? (Y/N)	
Comparator(s)	
Outcomes	
Statistically significant?	
Clinically significant?	
Side effects observed	
Safety issues, if any	
Did the study population represent YOU (age, gender, ethnicity, etc.)?	
In your judgment, does this study support you taking this product? Why or why not?	

THE 95% VEGAN DIET WORKBOOK

Complete the following checklist for each study published.

Study Title:	
Study sponsor(s):	
Human population:	
Average age of study subjects:	
Age range:	
Both genders equally? (Y/N)	
Race/ethnicities studied	
Number of study subjects (people)	
Statistical powering %:	
Length of study:	
Study design: parallel? crossover?	
Double-blind?	
Prospective? (Y/N)	
Randomized? (Y/N)	
What controls were in place?	
Hypothesis stated? (Y/N)	
Comparator(s)	
Outcomes	
Statistically significant?	
Clinically significant?	
Side effects observed	
Safety issues, if any	
Did the study population represent YOU (age, gender, ethnicity, etc.)?	
In your judgment, does this study support you taking this product? Why or why not?	

Complete the following checklist for each study published.

Study Title:	
Study sponsor(s):	
Human population:	
Average age of study subjects:	
Age range:	
Both genders equally? (Y/N)	
Race/ethnicities studied	
Number of study subjects (people)	
Statistical powering %:	
Length of study:	
Study design: parallel? crossover?	
Double-blind?	
Prospective? (Y/N)	
Randomized? (Y/N)	
What controls were in place?	
Hypothesis stated? (Y/N)	
Comparator(s)	
Outcomes	
Statistically significant?	
Clinically significant?	
Side effects observed	
Safety issues, if any	
Did the study population represent YOU (age, gender, ethnicity, etc.)?	
In your judgment, does this study support you taking this product? Why or why not?	

THE 95% VEGAN DIET WORKBOOK

Good Science Checklist	
Product name:	
Number of studies completed in humans:	
Studies published in:	
Journal:	
Journal:	
Journal:	
Journal:	
Journal:	

Complete the following checklist for each study published.

Study Title:	
Study sponsor(s):	
Human population:	
Average age of study subjects:	
Age range:	
Both genders equally? (Y/N)	
Race/ethnicities studied	
Number of study subjects (people)	
Statistical powering %:	
Length of study:	
Study design: parallel? crossover?	
Double-blind?	
Prospective? (Y/N)	
Randomized? (Y/N)	
What controls were in place?	
Hypothesis stated? (Y/N)	
Comparator(s)	
Outcomes	
Statistically significant?	
Clinically significant?	
Side effects observed	
Safety issues, if any	
Did the study population represent YOU (age, gender, ethnicity, etc.)?	
In your judgment, does this study support you taking this product? Why or why not?	

Complete the following checklist for each study published.

Study Title:	
Study sponsor(s):	
Human population:	
Average age of study subjects:	
Age range:	
Both genders equally? (Y/N)	
Race/ethnicities studied	
Number of study subjects (people)	
Statistical powering %:	
Length of study:	
Study design: parallel? crossover?	
Double-blind?	
Prospective? (Y/N)	
Randomized? (Y/N)	
What controls were in place?	
Hypothesis stated? (Y/N)	
Comparator(s)	
Outcomes	
Statistically significant?	
Clinically significant?	
Side effects observed	
Safety issues, if any	
Did the study population represent YOU (age, gender, ethnicity, etc.)?	
In your judgment, does this study support you taking this product? Why or why not?	

THE 95% VEGAN DIET WORKBOOK

Complete the following checklist for each study published.

Study Title:	
Study sponsor(s):	
Human population:	
Average age of study subjects:	
Age range:	
Both genders equally? (Y/N)	
Race/ethnicities studied	
Number of study subjects (people)	
Statistical powering %:	
Length of study:	
Study design: parallel? crossover?	
Double-blind?	
Prospective? (Y/N)	
Randomized? (Y/N)	
What controls were in place?	
Hypothesis stated? (Y/N)	
Comparator(s)	
Outcomes	
Statistically significant?	
Clinically significant?	
Side effects observed	
Safety issues, if any	
Did the study population represent YOU (age, gender, ethnicity, etc.)?	
In your judgment, does this study support you taking this product? Why or why not?	

Complete the following checklist for each study published.

Study Title:	
Study sponsor(s):	
Human population:	
Average age of study subjects:	
Age range:	
Both genders equally? (Y/N)	
Race/ethnicities studied	
Number of study subjects (people)	
Statistical powering %:	
Length of study:	
Study design: parallel? crossover?	
Double-blind?	
Prospective? (Y/N)	
Randomized? (Y/N)	
What controls were in place?	
Hypothesis stated? (Y/N)	
Comparator(s)	
Outcomes	
Statistically significant?	
Clinically significant?	
Side effects observed	
Safety issues, if any	
Did the study population represent YOU (age, gender, ethnicity, etc.)?	
In your judgment, does this study support you taking this product? Why or why not?	

Complete the following checklist for each study published.

Study Title:	
Study sponsor(s):	
Human population:	
Average age of study subjects:	
Age range:	
Both genders equally? (Y/N)	
Race/ethnicities studied	
Number of study subjects (people)	
Statistical powering %:	
Length of study:	
Study design: parallel? crossover?	
Double-blind?	
Prospective? (Y/N)	
Randomized? (Y/N)	
What controls were in place?	
Hypothesis stated? (Y/N)	
Comparator(s)	
Outcomes	
Statistically significant?	
Clinically significant?	
Side effects observed	
Safety issues, if any	
Did the study population represent YOU (age, gender, ethnicity, etc.)?	
In your judgment, does this study support you taking this product? Why or why not?	

Good Science Checklist	
Product name:	
Number of studies completed in humans:	
Studies published in:	
Journal:	
Journal:	
Journal:	
Journal:	
Journal:	

Complete the following checklist for each study published.

Study Title:	
Study sponsor(s):	
Human population:	
Average age of study subjects:	
Age range:	
Both genders equally? (Y/N)	
Race/ethnicities studied	
Number of study subjects (people)	
Statistical powering %:	
Length of study:	
Study design: parallel? crossover?	
Double-blind?	
Prospective? (Y/N)	
Randomized? (Y/N)	
What controls were in place?	
Hypothesis stated? (Y/N)	
Comparator(s)	
Outcomes	
Statistically significant?	
Clinically significant?	
Side effects observed	
Safety issues, if any	
Did the study population represent YOU (age, gender, ethnicity, etc.)?	
In your judgment, does this study support you taking this product? Why or why not?	

THE 95% VEGAN DIET WORKBOOK

Complete the following checklist for each study published.

Study Title:	
Study sponsor(s):	
Human population:	
Average age of study subjects:	
Age range:	
Both genders equally? (Y/N)	
Race/ethnicities studied	
Number of study subjects (people)	
Statistical powering %:	
Length of study:	
Study design: parallel? crossover?	
Double-blind?	
Prospective? (Y/N)	
Randomized? (Y/N)	
What controls were in place?	
Hypothesis stated? (Y/N)	
Comparator(s)	
Outcomes	
Statistically significant?	
Clinically significant?	
Side effects observed	
Safety issues, if any	
Did the study population represent YOU (age, gender, ethnicity, etc.)?	
In your judgment, does this study support you taking this product? Why or why not?	

Complete the following checklist for each study published.

Study Title:	
Study sponsor(s):	
Human population:	
Average age of study subjects:	
Age range:	
Both genders equally? (Y/N)	
Race/ethnicities studied	
Number of study subjects (people)	
Statistical powering %:	
Length of study:	
Study design: parallel? crossover?	
Double-blind?	
Prospective? (Y/N)	
Randomized? (Y/N)	
What controls were in place?	
Hypothesis stated? (Y/N)	
Comparator(s)	
Outcomes	
Statistically significant?	
Clinically significant?	
Side effects observed	
Safety issues, if any	
Did the study population represent YOU (age, gender, ethnicity, etc.)?	
In your judgment, does this study support you taking this product? Why or why not?	

THE 95% VEGAN DIET WORKBOOK

Complete the following checklist for each study published.

Study Title:	
Study sponsor(s):	
Human population:	
Average age of study subjects:	
Age range:	
Both genders equally? (Y/N)	
Race/ethnicities studied	
Number of study subjects (people)	
Statistical powering %:	
Length of study:	
Study design: parallel? crossover?	
Double-blind?	
Prospective? (Y/N)	
Randomized? (Y/N)	
What controls were in place?	
Hypothesis stated? (Y/N)	
Comparator(s)	
Outcomes	
Statistically significant?	
Clinically significant?	
Side effects observed	
Safety issues, if any	
Did the study population represent YOU (age, gender, ethnicity, etc.)?	
In your judgment, does this study support you taking this product? Why or why not?	

Complete the following checklist for each study published.

Study Title:	
Study sponsor(s):	
Human population:	
Average age of study subjects:	
Age range:	
Both genders equally? (Y/N)	
Race/ethnicities studied	
Number of study subjects (people)	
Statistical powering %:	
Length of study:	
Study design: parallel? crossover?	
Double-blind?	
Prospective? (Y/N)	
Randomized? (Y/N)	
What controls were in place?	
Hypothesis stated? (Y/N)	
Comparator(s)	
Outcomes	
Statistically significant?	
Clinically significant?	
Side effects observed	
Safety issues, if any	
Did the study population represent YOU (age, gender, ethnicity, etc.)?	
In your judgment, does this study support you taking this product? Why or why not?	

Good Science Checklist	
Product name:	
Number of studies completed in humans:	
Studies published in:	
Journal:	
Journal:	
Journal:	
Journal:	
Journal:	

Complete the following checklist for each study published.

Study Title:	
Study sponsor(s):	
Human population:	
Average age of study subjects:	
Age range:	
Both genders equally? (Y/N)	
Race/ethnicities studied	
Number of study subjects (people)	
Statistical powering %:	
Length of study:	
Study design: parallel? crossover?	
Double-blind?	
Prospective? (Y/N)	
Randomized? (Y/N)	
What controls were in place?	
Hypothesis stated? (Y/N)	
Comparator(s)	
Outcomes	
Statistically significant?	
Clinically significant?	
Side effects observed	
Safety issues, if any	
Did the study population represent YOU (age, gender, ethnicity, etc.)?	
In your judgment, does this study support you taking this product? Why or why not?	

Complete the following checklist for each study published.

Study Title:	
Study sponsor(s):	
Human population:	
Average age of study subjects:	
Age range:	
Both genders equally? (Y/N)	
Race/ethnicities studied	
Number of study subjects (people)	
Statistical powering %:	
Length of study:	
Study design: parallel? crossover?	
Double-blind?	
Prospective? (Y/N)	
Randomized? (Y/N)	
What controls were in place?	
Hypothesis stated? (Y/N)	
Comparator(s)	
Outcomes	
Statistically significant?	
Clinically significant?	
Side effects observed	
Safety issues, if any	
Did the study population represent YOU (age, gender, ethnicity, etc.)?	
In your judgment, does this study support you taking this product? Why or why not?	

THE 95% VEGAN DIET WORKBOOK

Complete the following checklist for each study published.

Study Title:	
Study sponsor(s):	
Human population:	
Average age of study subjects:	
Age range:	
Both genders equally? (Y/N)	
Race/ethnicities studied	
Number of study subjects (people)	
Statistical powering %:	
Length of study:	
Study design: parallel? crossover?	
Double-blind?	
Prospective? (Y/N)	
Randomized? (Y/N)	
What controls were in place?	
Hypothesis stated? (Y/N)	
Comparator(s)	
Outcomes	
Statistically significant?	
Clinically significant?	
Side effects observed	
Safety issues, if any	
Did the study population represent YOU (age, gender, ethnicity, etc.)?	
In your judgment, does this study support you taking this product? Why or why not?	

Complete the following checklist for each study published.

Study Title:	
Study sponsor(s):	
Human population:	
Average age of study subjects:	
Age range:	
Both genders equally? (Y/N)	
Race/ethnicities studied	
Number of study subjects (people)	
Statistical powering %:	
Length of study:	
Study design: parallel? crossover?	
Double-blind?	
Prospective? (Y/N)	
Randomized? (Y/N)	
What controls were in place?	
Hypothesis stated? (Y/N)	
Comparator(s)	
Outcomes	
Statistically significant?	
Clinically significant?	
Side effects observed	
Safety issues, if any	
Did the study population represent YOU (age, gender, ethnicity, etc.)?	
In your judgment, does this study support you taking this product? Why or why not?	

Complete the following checklist for each study published.

Study Title:	
Study sponsor(s):	
Human population:	
Average age of study subjects:	
Age range:	
Both genders equally? (Y/N)	
Race/ethnicities studied	
Number of study subjects (people)	
Statistical powering %:	
Length of study:	
Study design: parallel? crossover?	
Double-blind?	
Prospective? (Y/N)	
Randomized? (Y/N)	
What controls were in place?	
Hypothesis stated? (Y/N)	
Comparator(s)	
Outcomes	
Statistically significant?	
Clinically significant?	
Side effects observed	
Safety issues, if any	
Did the study population represent YOU (age, gender, ethnicity, etc.)?	
In your judgment, does this study support you taking this product? Why or why not?	

DIET, SUPPLEMENTS, YOUR PRESCRIPTION, AND OVER-THE-COUNTER MEDICATION

To say that there are far too many medicines, supplements, and foods to keep track of all of the potential interactions is a gross understatement. While many of these interactions are fairly well known, it is likely that many more have not yet been identified. In that we can only work with the information available, we will never get it all perfect. However, because of the possible combinations and the unlikelihood that all potential interactions will be spotted by your healthcare provider(s), it is of utmost importance that you stay on top of everything you take and how it may interact with other drugs, supplements, and foods.

Medication/Supplement	Strength	Dosage (1 tablet/cap-sule, 2 tablet/ capsules, etc.)	How many times do you take it per day?	What do you take it for?	Prescription or over-the-counter?	Prescribing healthcare provider/ specialty
Example: Lisinopril	20mg	1 tablet	once	High blood pressure	Prescription	Dr. Smith/ Internist

CREATE A RIPPLE EFFECT

Creating a ripple effect for the generations to come will not happen by accident. We all need to intentionally incorporate actions into our daily lives that will positively impact others. Here we will share our first ten guidelines to get you thinking about how all of this applies in your life. Then you will be provided a means by which you can plan to create a ripple effect for your family, friends, and community.

THE FIRST TEN GUIDELINES TO CREATE A RIPPLE EFFECT, GENERATION TO GENERATION

1. Make the nutrition of your family a priority. Keep your vision for creating a nutritionally healthy environment top of mind for your kids. This will teach them that their health is something to be respected and cherished.

2. Make the physical activity of your family a priority. You don't need a gym membership to ensure your family is getting enough exercise. Play outside with your kids, jump rope, play tag, or whatever your child's preference. Take a stroll around the block with your kids when you all get home for the day. If you can't get outside where you live to exercise, explore what may be available in your community for you and your kids to do. This will allow your kids to tell you about their day at the same time you are all getting some exercise in.

3. Teach your kids how to fish. Create a poster board for a daily nutrition roundup that actively engages them. However you choose to do it, help them understand the importance of keeping their fat and animal protein intake low.

4. Take your kids to the supermarket or farmer's market and involve them in the selection of fresh fruits, vegetables, and whole grains. Encourage them to choose all of the different food colors so that they have a varied diet. If the fresh whole food is too expensive, take them over to the freezer section and select some less pricey options. Help them understand why choices are good or not. For example, is it too high in fat and too low in fiber? Does the food contain animal products?

185

5. Do not reward your kids with food. I cringe when I hear parents promising some fattening treat (such as a candy bar or ice cream) as a reward. Your kids will value even more highly rewards that involve spending time together doing something they will enjoy. For example, when your child brings home that A+ test, why not celebrate with a trip to the nearest playground? This will also give them and you some much needed exercise.

6. Remember you are in charge of your own wallet. If your kids beg you for an unhealthy fast-food meal, you do have a choice. Perhaps you can get them to think about how that money could be better spent while reminding them the reasons why they are not going to eat that unhealthy meal. You might even start saving the money you would have spent in a jar at home and ultimately spend it on something much more enjoyable for the whole family. It is always good to give your kids a visual when trying to teach them a principle.

7. Do not offer second helpings. We already eat far too much. Help your kids understand what a healthy portion size looks like and tell them when they have had enough. This is just a boundary that children need to learn so that they will carry it through to adulthood.

8. Teach your children that it is okay to be hungry. For some reason, we have gotten to the point in our society where we think any pangs of hunger are unacceptable when in fact they are normal. Think about how often you eat when you are not even hungry. Yes, there is a psychological component to feeling hungry, such as smelling food or seeing a commercial that makes your kids want to run out and grab that huge steak burger. This is another boundary that is healthy for children to learn: to have the self-discipline out of respect for their health to not succumb to the temptation to gorge themselves.

9. Minimize trips to the local fast-food restaurants. Although some of them are trying to convince you they have healthier options, often times they are adding items that may be a bit lower in fat (still too high in some cases) but have large quantities of simple sugars. In short, not healthy options.

10. Address it quickly if your kids start to head down the wrong nutritional path. If they are being influenced by other kids to make unhealthy food or dietary habit choices, remind them of what they learned when they were out grocery shopping with you, as well as all of the other lessons you have weaved into their minds.

Above all this, *you* must become a role model for your children; *you* must also follow these guidelines. And as you incorporate these ten guidelines into your family's reality, you will come across so many best practices. Be sure to share them with others in your community and also learn from them. This is how we will find our way out of this unhealthy mess we have allowed to take over, by creating a ripple effect throughout our communities as well as from generation to generation!

YOUR PLAN FOR CREATING A RIPPLE EFFECT

Insert your plans, and then stick to them!

Person(s)	Occasion	Action(s)	Due date	Outcome	Follow-up steps
Example: Jenny (daughter)	Grocery shopping	Have her choose fresh vegetables	January 3, 2014	She learned the importance of choosing a variety of colors for good nutrition	Next, have her choose fruit to make smoothies and popsicles - make together as a family

YOUR PLAN FOR CREATING A RIPPLE EFFECT

Person(s)	Occasion	Action(s)	Due date	Outcome	Follow-up steps

QUIT SMOKING

As you may recall from the book, the most important thing you can do for your health is to quit smoking, if you do smoke. All of the good nutrition and medicine in the world cannot outweigh the damages to your health that smoking causes.

To help you move forward, here we provide the Standard of Care from Smokefree.gov, created by the Tobacco Control Research Branch of the National Cancer Institute (http://www.smokefree.gov/).

OVERVIEW OF THE BASIC STEPS TO PREPARE TO QUIT

The National Cancer Institute (NCI) recommends how to prepare to quit smoking through the acronym START. START stands for:

S = Set a quit date.

T = Tell family, friends, and coworkers that you plan to quit.

A = Anticipate and plan for the challenges you'll face while quitting.

R = Remove cigarettes and other tobacco products from your home, car, and work.

T = Talk to your doctor about getting help to quit.

SET A QUIT DATE

In setting a quit date, NCI recommends picking a day within the next two weeks so that you have time to prepare but do not lose motivation from waiting too long. NCI also recommends quitting on a weekend so that you have a jumpstart on quitting when the work week starts.

TELL FAMILY, FRIENDS, AND COWORKERS ABOUT PLANS TO QUIT

NCI recommends telling those around you about your plans to quit smoking, as well as giving them some specific instructions on how they can help you, including:

- Whether or not you will want to discuss how you are doing,

- Asking them to understand and be patient with any mood changes for a couple of weeks after you quit, and

- If someone you know smokes, asking them not to smoke around you or even join you in quitting.

Asking for support from people in your life and finding support groups in person or even online is absolutely okay. There is no shame in asking for help, especially when quitting smoking is so crucial to your long-term health! Your state has a toll-free telephone quit line. Call 1-800-QUIT-NOW (1-800-784-8669) to get one-on-one help quitting, support and coping strategies, and referrals to resources and local cessation programs. You can also visit the National Cancer Institute's smokefree.gov web site at http://www.smokefree.gov or contact NCI's smoking quitline at 1-877-44U-QUIT. Smokefree.gov offers science-driven tools, information, and support that has helped smokers quit. You will find state and national resources, free materials, and quitting advice from the National Cancer Institute and its partners.

ANTICIPATE AND PLAN FOR CHALLENGES

Quitting smoking is not easy, and you are going to encounter temptations and cravings, but if you can anticipate and plan for them, you are more likely to be successful. One resource available at Smokefree.gov is a craving journal, which can help you with this. Writing out a plan for how you will handle cravings will give you better chance of being successful.

REMOVE CIGARETTES AND OTHER TOBACCO PRODUCTS FROM YOUR HOME, CAR, AND WORK

Along with getting rid of all tobacco products, ashtrays, and other tobacco paraphernalia, NCI recommends getting rid of things that remind you of smoking. This includes scents! You should get your home, car, and work environment as clean and fresh-smelling as possible, maybe even getting candles and incense to mask any old smoke smell. You should also get your teeth cleaned by a dentist to get rid of smoking stains and residual taste. Finally, do not switch from one form of tobacco to another; they are all harmful to your health.

TALK TO YOUR DOCTOR ABOUT GETTING HELP TO QUIT

Your doctor is your health partner; talk to him or her about quitting smoking. He or she can recommend over-the-counter and prescription medications to help you cope with withdrawal symptoms. If you cannot talk with a doctor, there are over-the-counter products available at your local drugstore to help you quit, such as the nicotine patch and nicotine gum. A pharmacist can help you determine which product is right for you. If you are pregnant or plan to become pregnant, you should talk with a doctor before starting any medication.

Another thing NCI recommends is to speak with your doctor and pharmacist about your quitting smoking, citing that nicotine affects how some drugs work which may require some adjustment of your medications.

On your first smoke-free day, you should remind people around you that it is your quit date and ask them to be supportive. NCI also recommends that when you actually quit, you should use your support program (official or self-made) as much and as often as you need and keep busy (maybe start a new hobby) so that you do not fixate on smoking. Also, ask your support partners to help you stay away from temptations that make you think about smoking.

If you are using a medication to help you quit, then follow its directions. Do not rush to wean yourself off the medication; twelve weeks is usually a good minimum for using cessation medication, but of course, listen to your doctor if he says otherwise in your situation.

Smoking often includes a manual and oral fixation. When you quit smoking, you may find yourself feeling the need to hold something in your hand or mouth. NCI recommends holding a pencil, marble, paperclip, or other small object in your hand. If you miss having something in your mouth, try toothpicks, cinnamon sticks, lollipops, hard candy, sugar-free gum, or carrot sticks. Just also be careful that you do not replace smoking with excessive eating; people often gain weight when they quit. Remember that quitting smoking is not easy and that there are going to be temptations and cravings. That is why the "anticipate" part of START is very important, as is having a written plan of how you are going to handle cravings. Stick to what you wrote, or modify it slightly if you realize it was not realistic. But no matter what, do not give in to the temptation to have *just one*. Cigarettes are like potato chips, you can intend to have just one and slip to having two, three, or a dozen. You have worked hard to get to this point, and you do not want to undo all of your hard work by having even one cigarette! That said, if you do slip and have one cigarette, it does not make you a bad or weak person. That is The Guilt Factor trying to convince you that you should give up on quitting. Get back on the proverbial horse, reach out to your family and group support, and move on down the road to being smoke-free.

When things get difficult, also keep in mind the short- and long-term health benefits of quitting. In the short-term, your senses of smell and taste improve, you can breathe more easily, and your smoker's cough will start to get better. Over the long-term, you are reducing your risk of heart disease, stroke, chronic bronchitis, emphysema, and many kinds of cancer. You will also reduce your loved ones' exposure to second-hand smoke and set a better example for younger family members. Finally, with the money you save from not smoking, you can save up for a special reward for yourself! If you had a pack-a-day habit costing roughly $5 a day, that is $1,825 saved in just one year! Think of all the great things you could do with that kind of money.

There are many good reasons to quit smoking, but one that we have not mentioned yet is the sense of personal pride that you should (and will) have at accomplishing this goal. It may not be an easy task, but you will find that your efforts are richly rewarded with better health, saving money, and a general sense of well-being!

NOTES

NOTES

NOTES

NOTES

NOTES

NOTES

NOTES

NOTES

NOTES

NOTES

NOTES

NOTES

NOTES

NOTES

NOTES

NOTES

NOTES

NOTES

NOTES

NOTES

REFERENCES

THE IMPORTANCE OF LEARNING HOW TO FISH

1. www.brookes.ac.uk/services/ocsd, June 27, 2002.

HOME-BASED ASSESSMENTS FOR NUTRITIONAL HEALTH STATUS

1. Eric J. Jacobs, et al., "Waist Circumference and All-Cause Mortality in a Large U.S. Cohort," *Arch Intern Med 2010* 170 (15) (2010): 1293–1301.

2. Ian Janssen, Peter Katzmarzyk, and Robert Ross, "Body Mass Index, Waist Circumference, and Health Risk, Evidence in Support of Current National Institutes of Health Guidelines," *Arch Intern Med* 162 (2002): 2074–2079.

3. http://www.nlm.nih.gov/medlineplus/ency/article/002222.htm

4. Michael F. Holick and Tai C. Chen, "Vitamin D Deficiency: A Worldwide Problem with Health Consequences, *Am J Clin Nutrition* 87 (suppl) (2008):1080S–6S.

5. Thomas J. Wang et al., "Vitamin D Deficiency and Risk of Cardiovascular Disease," *Circulation* 117 (2008): 503–511.

6. "NCEP Report: Implications of Recent Clinical Trials for the National Cholesterol Education Program Adult Treatment Panel III Guidelines." Available at http://www.nhlbi.nih.gov/guidelines/cholesterol/atp3upd04.pdf.

7. Paul S. Jellinger et al., "American Association of Clinical Endocrinologists' Guidelines for Management of Dyslipidemia and Prevention of Atherosclerosis," *Endocrine Practice* 18 (Suppl 1) (March/April 2012).

8. Sabine Kahl and Michael Roden, "An Update on the Pathogenesis of Type 2 Diabetes Mellitus," *Hamdan Medical Journal 2012* 5 (2012): 99–122.

9. Terry W. Du Clos, "Function of C-Reactive Protein," *Annals of Medicine* 32, no. 4 (2000): 274–278.

10. Paul M. Ridker, Robert J. Glynn, and Charles H. Hennekens, "C-Reactive Protein Adds to the Predictive Value of Total and HDL Cholesterol in Determining Risk of First Myocardial Infarction," *Circulation* 97 (1998): 2007–2011.

11. Paul M. Ridker et al., "Prospective Study of C-Reactive Protein and the Risk of Future Cardiovascular Events Among Apparently Healthy Women," *Circulation* 98 (1998): 731–733

12. Katherine Esposito et al., "Effect of a Mediterranean-Style Diet on Endothelial Dysfunction and Markers of Vascular Inflammation in the Metabolic Syndrome," *JAMA* 292, no. 12 (Sept 22/29, 2004): 1440–1446.

13. David J.A. Jenkins et al., "Effects of a Dietary Portfolio of Cholesterol-Lowering Foods vs Lovastatin on Serum Lipids and C-Reactive Protein," *JAMA* 290, no. 4 (July 23/30, 2003): 502–510.

14. Earl S. Ford, "Does Exercise Reduce Inflammation? Physical Activity and C-Reactive Protein Among U.S. Adults" (2002).

15. Steven E. Nissen et al., "Statin Therapy, LDL Cholesterol, C-Reactive Protein, and Coronary Artery Disease," *New England Journal of Medicine 2005* 352 (2005): 29–38.

16. Richard M. Green and Steven Flamm, "AGA Technical Review on the Evaluation of Liver Chemistry Tests," *Gastroenterology* 123, 4 (October 2002): 1367–1384.

THE MACRONUTRIENTS: CARBOHYDRATE, FAT, AND PROTEIN

1. J. Salmeron et al., "Dietary Fiber, Glycemic Load, and Risk of Non-Insulin-Dependent Diabetes Mellitus in Women," *JAMA* 277 (1997): 472–477.

2. Wayne W. Campbell et al., "Dietary Protein Requirements of Younger and Older Adults," *Am. J. Clin. Nutr. 2008* 88 (2008): 1322–1329.

3. Mohammad A. Humayun et al., "Reevaluation of the Protein Requirement in Young Men with the Indicator Amino Acid Oxidation Technique," *Am. J. Clin. Nutr.* 86 (2007): 995–1002.

4. Douglas Paddon-Jones et al., "Role of Dietary Protein in the Sarcopenia of Aging," *Am. J. Clin. Nutr.* 87 (suppl) (2008): 1562S–1566S.

5. Jane E. Kerstetter et al., "Dietary Protein Affects Intestinal Calcium Absorption, *Am. J. Clin. Nutr.* 68 (1998): 859–865.

6. Marian T. Hannan et al., "Effect of Dietary Protein on Bone Loss in Elderly Men and Women: The Framingham Osteoporosis Study," *Journal of Bone and Mineral Research* 15, no. 12 (2000): 2504–2512.

7. William M. Rand et al., "Meta-Analysis of Nitrogen Balance Studies for Estimating Protein Requirements in Healthy Adults," *Am. J. Clin. Nutr.* 77 (2003): 109–127.

8. Vernon R. Young and Peter L. Pellet, "Plant Proteins in Relation to Human Protein and Amino Acid Nutrition," *Am. J. Clin. Nutr.* 59 (Suppl) (1994): 1203S–1212S.

9. J. L. Slavin, "Position of the American Dietetic Association: Health Implications of Dietary Fiber," *Journal of the American Dietetic Association* 108 (10) (2008): 1716–1731.

INDEX

A

A1c 25, 26, 28, 29, 30, 31, 32, 33, 34, 35, 36, 37
Albumin 22, 23
Alcohol 25, 26
Amino acids 22, 23, 43, 44, 121
Anemia 22, 28, 29, 30, 31, 32, 33, 34, 35, 36, 37
Animal 43, 185
Apples 55, 77
Apricots 67
Arrhythmias 23
Artichokes 55, 77
Arugula 67, 77, 89
Asian 77
Asparagus 55
Assessments 7, 9, 15, 21, 213
Atherosclerosis 213
Autoimmune 26
Avocados 55, 67, 77

B

Beans 43, 44, 55, 67, 77, 89
Beets 67, 77, 89
Blackberries 67, 77, 123
Blood 21, 22, 23, 24, 25, 26, 27, 89, 127, 184
Blood pressure 24, 184
Blueberries 67, 123
BMI 15, 16, 17, 18, 42, 121
Body fat 18
Bone 23, 42
Boysenberries 67
Bread 123
Breakfast 125, 126
Breast 16, 23
Broccoli 55, 67, 77, 89
Brussels sprouts 55, 77, 89
Burdock 77

C

Cabbage 55, 67, 77, 89
Calcium 214
Calcium Absorption 214
Calories 42, 121, 122, 123, 124
Cancer 189, 190
Cancers 21
Carb 40, 41
Carbohydrate 25, 39, 122, 123, 124
Cardiovascular Disease 213
Carrots 67, 77, 89
Cauliflower 55, 67, 77, 89
CBC (Complete Blood Count) 21, 28, 29, 30, 31, 32, 33, 34, 35, 36, 37
CDC (Centers for Disease Control) 15, 16, 46
Celery 55, 67, 77, 89
Chard 55, 89
Cherries 55, 67
Chinese 8, 13, 100
Cholesterol 24, 213, 214
Christmas 8, 94
Chromium 45, 46
Cigarette 24, 191
Cinco De Mayo 8, 64
Citrons 89
Clean 15 51
Clinical 21
Cockgroft-Gault 22
Collards 55, 77, 89
Colonoscopies 21
Condiment 122, 125
Constipation 22
Contaminants 45, 46
Contamination 46
Controlled 25
Cooking 4

Corn 67, 77
Cravings 190, 191
C-Reactive Protein (CRP) - Chronic Elevation 21, 26
Cream 186
Creatinine 22, 23, 28, 29, 30, 31, 32, 33, 34, 35, 36, 37
Cucumbers 67, 77

D

Dairy 22, 53, 124
Dates 55, 67, 77
Dehydration 23
Dessert 122, 125
Diabetes 9, 26, 127, 213, 214
Diet 4, 9, 124, 183, 214
Dietary 24, 39, 44, 186
Disease 16, 21, 22, 23, 24, 25, 43, 191
Disinfectants 45
Drugs 25, 183, 190

E

Earth Day 7, 60
Easter 7, 62
Eggplant 67
Elderly 215
Electrocardiogram 21
Electron 4
Endive 77, 89
Environmental 45
EPA 45, 46
Ethnicity 18
Exercise 25, 109, 185, 186
Exposure 23, 191

F

Fasting 21, 23, 25
Fat 18, 19, 20, 24, 39, 42, 43, 121, 122, 123, 124, 185, 186
Fava beans 55, 89
Fennel 55, 77, 89
Ferritin 22
Fiber 7, 39, 40, 41, 49, 50, 214, 215
Figs 67, 77
Fish 13, 185
Flax Seed 123

Folic acid 21
Frugal 7, 55
Fruits 7, 8, 55, 67, 77, 89, 123, 124

G

Genetic 25
GFR 22
Ginger 67
Glycemic 39, 40
Google 47
Grain 122, 123, 125
Grandchildren 11
Grapefruit 55
Grapes 67, 77
Green beans 67, 77
Grocery shopping 186
Guavas 77, 89
Guilt Factor 191
Gym 185

H

Halloween 8, 84
Hanukkah 8, 92
HDL 23, 24, 25, 26, 28, 29, 30, 31, 32, 33, 34, 35, 36, 37, 214
Healthcare 11, 25, 26, 183, 184
Healthcare providers 11
Health Status 7, 9, 15, 21, 213
Heart disease 23, 191
Height 15, 22, 121
Hemoglobin 21, 22
Herbicides 51
Homework 11
Honey 124
Hunger 186
Hungry 186
Hydration 22
Hypertension 24

I

IBW 121
Ice cream 186
Iliac crests 15
Immune 21
Infection 21, 26

Insulin 214
Iron 11, 21, 22

J

Jicama 55, 77, 89

K

Kale 55, 77, 89
Kidney 22
Kiwi 77
Kumquats 55, 77
Kwanzaa 8, 96

L

Labor Day 8, 74
LDL 23, 24, 25, 26, 28, 29, 30, 31, 32, 33, 34, 35, 36,
    37, 43, 214
Leeks 55, 77, 89
Legume 122, 124, 125
Lemons 55, 67, 77, 89
Lettuce 55, 67, 77, 89
Limes 55, 77, 89
Lipid 28, 29, 30, 31, 32, 33, 34, 35, 36, 37
Literature 16
Liver 21, 23, 24, 26
Lysine 44, 121

M

Macronutrients 7, 9, 39, 214
Mammograms 21
Mandarin oranges 55, 77, 89
Maple syrup 124
Mardi Gras 8, 104
Medication 24
Melons 67
Meta-Analysis 215
Metabolism 23
Methionine 44
Milk 44
Minerals 46
Moderation 25
Molecular weight 45, 46
Mood 189
Mortality 213
Mother Cabrini 8, 72

Mulberries 67
Muscle 42, 123
Mushrooms 55, 77, 89

N

National Cancer Institute 189, 190
National Cholesterol Education Program 213
Nectarines 67, 77
New Year 8, 98, 100
NIH (National Institutes of Health) 116
Nitrogen 215
Non-dairy 124
Noodles 123
Note 18, 122
NSF 45, 46, 47
Nutrition 123, 185, 187, 189
Nutritional Health Status 7, 9, 15, 21, 213
Nutritional status 21, 26
Nutritional yeast flakes 43
Nuts 43

O

Obese 15
Obesity 15, 18, 24, 43
Oils 123
Okra 67, 77
Oktoberfest 8, 82
Olives 67
Onions 67, 77, 89
Orange juice 25
Oranges 55, 67, 77, 89
Organic 7, 39, 51
Osteoporosis 215
Overweight 15, 18, 23, 25

P

Pap smears 21
Parsnips 55, 77, 89
Pasta 123
Peaches 67, 77, 123
Peanuts 67, 89
Pears 67, 77
Peas 43, 67, 77
Pecans 77
Peppers 67, 77

Persimmons 77
Pesticides 45, 51
Pharmacist 190
Physical Activity 214
Physicians 11, 22, 25
Pistachios 77
Plaque 23
Plums 67, 77
Pluots 67
Pomegranates 77
Pomelos 55, 89
Popcorn 124
Portion Size 40, 41
Potatoes 44, 55, 77, 89
Pregnancy 23
Pretzels 124
Prevention 213
Prostate 21
Protein 21, 22, 23, 26, 39, 42, 43, 44, 121, 122, 123, 124, 185
Prunes 40
Psychological 186

Q

Quince 77

R

Radishes 55, 89
Raspberries 67, 77
Research 189, 215
Reverse osmosis 46, 47
Rhubarb 67, 77
Rice 123
Ripple Effect 9, 185, 187, 188
Role model 186
Rutabagas 89

S

Scallions 55
Science 9, 131, 132, 137, 142, 147, 152, 157, 162, 167, 172, 177
Scientific 24
Scientist 9, 131
Seasonal 7, 8, 55, 67, 77, 89
Sex 18
Shallots 55

Sleep 8, 109, 116, 117
Smoke 189, 190, 191
Soy 43, 44, 124
Spices 124
Spinach 67, 77, 89
Squash 44, 89
Statins 26
Steak 186
St. Patrick's Day 7, 58, 59
Strawberries 55, 67, 77, 123
Study Checklist 130-179
Sugar 21, 25, 40, 191
Summer 8, 67, 123
Sun exposure 23
Super Bowl Sunday 8, 102
Supermarket 185
Supplement 26, 184
Sweet potatoes 77, 89
Systematic 11

T

Tangerines 55
Tayberries 67
Tempeh 123
Thanksgiving 8, 86
The Guilt Factor 8
Thyroid 21, 23
Tobacco 189, 190
Tofu 43
Tomatoes 67
Toxic 45
Transferrin 22
Triglyceride 23, 25
Turnips 55, 77, 89
TVP – Texturized Vegetable Protein 124

U

Umbilicus 15
Urinalysis 21, 27
Urine 21

V

Valentine's Day 8, 106
Vegan 21, 22, 23, 26, 39, 43, 53, 55, 121, 122
Vegetables 7, 8, 55, 67, 77, 89, 123, 124
Very Low Density Lipoprotein (VLDL) 25

Vitamin 21, 23, 28, 29, 30, 31, 32, 33, 34, 35, 36, 37, 213

W

Waist 16, 17, 18, 213
Walnuts 77
Water 7, 39, 45, 46
Weight 8, 42, 43, 121, 122
Whole food 185
Whole grains 185
Wine 25

Y

Yeast 124
Yogurt 123